Irritable Lower Syndrome & Giardia

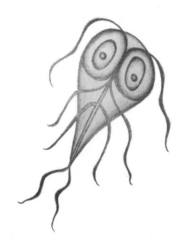

Irritable Bowel Syndrome & Giardia

– a parasite associated with IBS, gallbladder disease and other health issues

Susan Koten
MNIMH, MRCHM

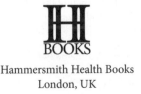

Hammersmith Health Books
London, UK

First published in 2019 by Hammersmith Health Books – an imprint of
Hammersmith Books Limited
4/4A Bloomsbury Square, London WC1A 2RP, UK
www.hammersmithbooks.co.uk

The information contained in this book is for educational purposes only. It is
the result of the study and the experience of the author. Whilst the information
and advice offered are believed to be true and accurate at the time of going to
press, neither the author nor the publisher can accept any legal responsibility or
liability for any errors or omissions that may have been made or for any adverse
effects which may occur as a result of following the recommendations given
herein. Always consult a qualified medical practitioner if you have any concerns
regarding your health.

British Library Cataloguing in Publication Data: A CIP record of this book is
available from the British Library.

Print ISBN 978-1-78161-100-5
Ebook ISBN 978-1-78161-101-2

Commissioning editor: Georgina Bentliff
Designed and typeset by: Julie Bennett of Bespoke Publishing Ltd.
Cover design by: Nicola Koten and Stuart Doyle
Cover photograph: © B-D-S Piotr Marcinski/shutterstock.com
Index: Dr Laurence Errington
Production: Helen Whitehorn, Pathmedia Ltd.
Printed and bound by: TJ International Ltd, Cornwall, UK
Giardia illustration: Amanda Humphries

Contents

Acknowledgements	*viii*
Preface	*ix*
Introduction	*xiii*
About the author	*xvi*
Chapter 1: What is Giardia?	**1**
Recognising symptoms	4
Laura's story	5
The life cycle of Giardia	7
Stage 1 Trophozoite (feeding) stage	7
Stage 2 The cyst stage	9
Travellers, beware!	10
Celia's story	10
Julia's story	11
Chapter 2: Getting a diagnosis	**14**
Rachel's story	15
Testing for Giardia	15
Stool ova and parasite (O&P) tests	16
ELISA stool test	16
String test	16
Comprehensive parasitology stool test	16
Testing for irritable bowel syndrome (IBS)	17
Testing for inflammatory bowel disease (IBD)	18
Manual muscle testing	19
Sophie's story	22
Chapter 3: Checking for Giardia	**26**
Health checklist	31
Getting help	32
Sally's story	32
Chapter 4: Gut reactions	**34**
James's story	35

Coeliac disease   35
Penny's story   37
Lactose intolerance   38
Leaky gut syndrome and food allergies   39
Vitamin B12 deficiency   39
Mary's story   40
Chapter 5: Giardia and stress   **42**
Jane's story   42
So what is stress?   44
How the immune systems reacts to stress   45
Recognising symptoms of stress   46
Giardia feeds stress   48
Alison's story   50
Chapter 6: Giardia and our natural defence barriers **54**
The microbiome   54
The mucus barrier   54
Factors for a healthy gut flora composition   55
Formation of a healthy microbiome   56
Giardia in pregnancy   57
Giardia and children   58
Becky's story   59
Poor diet   61
Chapter 7: Allergies   **63**
Asthma   64
Tom's story   65
Allergic rhinitis   67
Allergies and the sinuses   68
Mould allergy   69
Food intolerances and allergies   69
Wheat allergy   70
Giardia and allergic skin problems   71
Urticaria   71
Angioedema   71
Maureen's story   72
Chapter 8: The gallbladder connection   **74**
The role of the gallbladder   75
Gallbladder removal – cholecystectomy   75
Gallbladder removal and Giardia   76
Carol's story   76
Gallbladder checklist   80

Chapter 9: The pancreas connection   **82**
Understanding the pancreas   84
Maintaining a healthy pancreas   84
Alice's story   85
Melanie's story   88
Chapter 10: Prevention   **92**
Proton pump inhibitors   96
Christopher's story   97
Understanding the risk   98
How Giardia gets into drinking water   99
What about my drinking water?   99
How can Giardia be removed from drinking water?   100
How can giardiasis be prevented?   100
Tony's story   103
Chapter 11: Treating giardiasis   **106**
The allopathic approach   107
    Metronidazole (Flagyl)   107
    Tinidazole (Tindamax)   108
    Quinacrine (Atabrine)   108
The malaria link   109
Sally's story   110
Treating Giardia with herbs   111
Infusion of dried *Artemisia annua*   112
Herbal sprays   113
Ann's story   114
Chapter 12: Healing through energy fields   **117**
The etheric body   119
David's story   120
The *chakras*   121
My sprays   123
How to use the sprays   124
Conclusion   125

Appendices   *127*
    Appendix I: Herbs   *129*
    Appendix II: Glossary of terms   *142*
    Appendix III: Living without gluten   *144*
    Appendix IV: Maintaining a healthy gut microbiome   *151*
References   *159*
Index   *168*

Acknowledgements

This book would never have been written without the help and support of family, friends, colleagues and patients, and I would like to express my deepest gratitude to everyone who has contributed towards its completion.

I am also greatly indebted to Linda Saunders for her time and effort in getting this book to its final stages.

My heartfelt thanks go to my two daughters who have stood by me and supported my efforts throughout.

Finally, my thoughts go to John and his contribution during the book's early stages of preparation, before he passed away.

Preface

In March 2010, Nikki Page came to my Clinic seeking help. Her story was particularly harrowing and her health issues were complex. Using my herbal remedies, I was able to help improve her situation and as a result of her experience, she wrote an article for the *Telegraph*. The article raised the public's awareness of the Giardia parasite and, because of its impact, I have been able to help many people recover their health from the ravages of a Giardia infestation, and some of their stories are in these pages.

I am indebted to Nikki for her contribution towards this book and this is her story.

Nikki's story

A stomach upset and a doctor's decision to treat it with a broad spectrum antibiotic changed my life. At 20 I was a fit, dynamic and very busy young woman. I don't even remember why I thought the stomach upset necessitated a visit to the doctor, but the consequences of that visit affected my entire life.

A few days later, I was spending the weekend with a friend in Surrey. My mouth started to ulcerate and strange marks began appearing on my skin. My friend took me to the local hospital clutching the Septrin I was taking. I was told that under no circumstances was I to stop taking the antibiotic and probably I'd eaten something that disagreed with me. Hours later, I couldn't eat or swallow fluids and my skin had started to ulcerate. My friend put me in his car and drove me to my doctor in London, who immediately had me admitted to hospital. By this time my eyes were bleeding and ulcers bulged under my

nails. I was ulcerated inside and out. I could no longer see. At
the hospital, calls were made to contact my family and bring
them to my bedside as it was realised I was suffering an extreme
reaction to the Septrin. Doctors and specialists went into
overdrive to save my sight and kidneys from permanent damage.

I was lucky; many others who have had similar reactions to
Septrin have died or suffered permanent organ damage. I had
survived. Some three weeks or so later, I was discharged from
hospital, still looking rather strange, and with many follow-up
appointments with specialists, but anticipating a full recovery.
I was told not to go into public places because, if I contracted
any infection, there was nothing they could do. I was told to rest
every day and to take a period of convalescence. Looking back,
I have no idea how I managed. I needed to work and wanted to
get on with my life and, seemingly, managed very well. Except
some things had changed dramatically.No one warned me of
any likely problems to follow.

No one suggested that rest and recuperation wouldn't be
enough. No one suggested that my gut would be completely
devoid of good bacteria or prone to all sorts of problems or
the ramifications of a poorly functioning dietary system. Of
course, this was many years ago, and I don't suppose they
knew what the repercussions were likely to be. Life was different
then: no dietary advice, no alternative medical guidance, no
supplements, no google!

And so it started: an almost permanently bloated stomach,
either constipation or diarrhoea, and debilitating wind as
constant companions, achy joints, inability to do any aerobic
exercise, but worst of all, dreadful fatigue that would just
overwhelm me.

Over the years, I went to doctors, endured deeply unpleasant
tests, visited specialists and desperately tried to lead a normal
life. It was extremely difficult, but I'm a very determined person!
I began to understand that certain foods and particular types
of exercise made me much worse. I read anything I could
find on alternative solutions since the medical profession had
failed me miserably, even suggesting at one point that it was
psychosomatic. To this day, I remember devouring and cutting
out every word that Hazel Courteney wrote in the first Alternative

Medicine column in the Sunday Times. It was as if someone had switched on the light.

My first real breakthrough came when I met a wonderful doctor who was a friend of my then husband's family, in Wichita, Kansas. Dr Riordan was a fully qualified doctor who specialised in developing alternative treatments for chronic illnesses; he was the first to identify the presence of parasites in my blood. With various treatments and a strict diet, he made my life bearable again.

At the time I first saw Dr Riordan, he ran tests which showed me reacting to over 50 of 80 basic foods. The problem was that if I stuck to the remaining 30 that I could eat, I would suddenly develop a sensitivity to one of them and have to stop eating it. Resting certain foods worked quite well, but there was no reliable way to know when I could and couldn't tolerate something, so eating was always difficult and eating out or at other people's houses a nightmare.

The stomach problems never went away. I just learned to control and live with them, but bad bouts would come back frequently. As well as the original symptoms, I suffered regularly from candida. In addition, I needed plenty of rest and endless supplements to lead a half-normal life. It's very easy to forget now that it is only recently that supermarkets and restaurants started to cater for those of us who have to watch what we eat.

Then just six years ago, I met Susan Koten. Gemma, a friend of mine recently back from India, had been diagnosed with giardiasis, a type of gastroenteritis caused by Giardia lamblia, a microscopic parasite which the World Health Organization classifies as one of the most common affecting humans. It can be transferred through polluted water or contact with animals, and reproduces in the small intestine

Gemma was loathe to take the prescribed antibiotics and had been introduced to Susan as a herbalist who had achieved particular success treating parasites. Gemma had exhibited so many symptoms I recognised that I too made an immediate appointment to see Susan.

And it is not over-exaggerating to say that appointment with Susan changed my life within days. I was indeed suffering from

Giardia. Her wormwood tonic proved almost magical in the way it turned my life around. My stomach calmed down almost immediately. I was able to add many things back into my diet. I could eat berries, which had hitherto caused too much acid in my system and almost instant joint pain. The results were truly amazing. My energy levels improved too.

I remain very prone to picking up any form of parasite and there are some things I know that I really must not eat (gluten, white potatoes (nightshade family), red meat, dairy except butter and, of course, too much sugar). Fortunately, they do not include chocolate! I have to work very hard at keeping my immune system strong and my gut really healthy. I have an incredibly healthy diet and I can tell the minute I get a bug in my stomach. But – and it's a huge but – I can eat healthy foods that I couldn't even look at before. I suffer far fewer bouts of stomach upsets. My skin is great and my energy levels are pretty good.

I am absolutely indebted to Susan for the relief her knowledge of parasites and the treatment of them has given me.

Introduction

Giardiasis has dominated my working life for the last 22 years. In that time, I have treated hundreds of patients whose debilitating digestive symptoms have disrupted their lives for many years, often leaving them with chronic ill health. I have listened to countless stories of visits to GPs, gastroenterologists, endless tests, only to have hopes of a recovery dashed when their intolerable symptoms return. By the time they reach me, patients are past 'desperate' and often don't know whether to resign themselves to a lifetime of health issues or to just try one last thing in the hope of finding a permanent solution to the problem. It is a 'what have I got to lose' situation, and they are thrilled when – sometimes within days – their symptoms clear up, and they feel better than they have for years.

Some already know, before they come to me, they have giardiasis. The diagnosis has been made, but conventional treatment has been ineffective. Others are struggling with what they believe to be IBS, although it is actually giardiasis.

From my years of treating this condition, it is clear to me that giardiasis is poorly understood, often misdiagnosed, and frequently mismanaged. So, what am I doing that others are not?

I have a special interest in Giardia – the parasite that causes giardiasis – and this started with my own experience, back in 1986. At the time I had just begun to train as a medical herbalist. I'd been fascinated by herbs since childhood, when I used to walk along the river banks looking at the thistles, burdock and other wild plants. I was now eager to turn my passion into a career that would help other people.

Following an overnight stay in hospital for a minor operation, I started to suffer from diarrhoea. At first I thought it was a passing bug and I would soon make a full recovery, but that wasn't to be the case. Various attempts to overcome the problem failed, and it started to affect my life completely. Any car journey was a nightmare, and my stress and anxiety levels rose as I tried to come to terms with the situation. The noises from my stomach were very disturbing, and so was the discomfort after eating. My weight dropped as I was unsure what I should eat, and the partially digested food shooting through my body was not staying long enough to give me the nourishment I needed.

I was in my first year of studies at the School of Herbal Medicine in Tunbridge Wells, and I also had two young children. The doctor said the cause was probably stress related and prescribed imodium but that, I felt, was only masking the problem.

I eventually decided I was not going to die from the condition and settled down to a bland diet of rice, fish and a few vegetables, and just carried on. I was not sufficiently knowledgeable in my chosen subject at the time to know how to treat myself.

I did consult the training clinic for herbal medicine and was given a herbal mixture which helped, but I felt it was not the complete cure. Something was wrong – but what? There is nothing like experiencing a problem to fully understand the implications of having it.

It was sometime after I qualified as a medical herbalist that I was drawn to an article in a herbal journal mentioning Giardia and bowel problems, which discussed a testing method using applied kinesiology. I booked myself on a course and started testing my patients for this parasite. This form of testing opened up a whole new dimension of locating the presence of Giardia very quickly and accurately.

It took many years of watching and treating my patients to get a clearer understanding of the effects of Giardia on the human body, the problems people faced using conventional treatment and the utter despair and desperation to find another method in order to get relief.

I have written this book so that anyone reading it who is suffering, or knows anyone suffering, from the symptoms of Giardia, may get help. Also, it is for any therapist who is seeing patients but maybe misdiagnosing this condition and not getting to the root cause. The protocol and techniques used are based on my own observations and experiences having seen many hundreds of patients suffering from digestive disorders over the last 20 years.

I cannot be certain that my own digestive issues were associated with Giardia as there was no one around to help me in this direction, or even suggest that this might be the cause of my problem. However, having experienced digestive problems made me understand the implications and misery that these can create and sent me on the journey to discover the cause.

To everyone who reads on, I hope this book will change your life for the better, in the same way my studies have changed mine.

About the Author

Susan Koten MNIMH, MRCHM is qualified in both Western and Chinese Herbal Medicine. She qualified as a Medical Herbalist in 1990 at the School of Herbal Medicine in Tunbridge Wells, UK. In 1997 she completed a course of clinical practice in Chinese Herbal Medicine at Nanjing International Acupuncture Training Centre in China and in 1998 completed a course at the School of Chinese Herbal Medicine under Michael McIntyre. She also qualified as a Bowen Technique Therapist in 1995 at the Bowen Therapy Academy in Australia. She is a Member of the National Institute of Medical Herbalists, a Member of the Register of Chinese Herbal Medicine, a Member of the British Institute for Allergy and Environmental Therapy and a Member of the Bowen Therapy Academy UK.

Chapter 1

What is Giardia?

As I sit down to write this book, the latest available statistics show that in 2016 there were 4492 recorded cases of Giardia infestation in England and Wales.[1] This figure has been steadily rising since 2007 and the World Health Organization estimates that 200 million people worldwide have symptoms of infection, with 500,000 new cases reported each year.[2]

Giardia is the parasite that causes the painful and debilitating gastric illness 'giardiasis'. It was first discovered in 1681 when the Dutch scientist Antony van Leeuwenhoek spotted it in a microscopic examination of his own stool, noting the organisms were around the size of a 'globule of blood' (that is, a red blood corpuscle as we would call it today).

Due to extremely poor sanitation, parasites were a universal problem at the time, and Leeuwenhoek had developed his own single lens microscope to discover more about them. Giardia would have looked a bit like a smiley face, with two eye-like nuclei peering out at him.

Nearly 200 years later, in 1859, the scientists Dr Vilem Dusan Lambi and Professor Alfred Giard added to Leeuwenhoek's work by formally describing the parasite's shape and size,[3] and, another 56 years later, in 1915, Charles Wardell Stiles gave it the name *Giardia lamblia*.

Other terms used are *Giardia intestinalis* or *Giardia duodenalis*,[4] which were added to the lexicon in the 1970s, after doctors linked the parasite to gastric illness in people who had travelled to parts of the world where Giardia was widespread.

Historians now believe that Giardia may have been one source of the intestinal illnesses that plagued the crusaders. The theory is backed up by archeological evidence of the parasite having colonised a mediaeval latrine in the crusader city of Acre.[5] Indeed, Giardia could have been the reason that King Louis IV was struck down so badly with diarrhoea while leading the Seventh Crusade in 1249 that, as legend has it, 'parts of his breeches had to be cut away'!

Giardia can live in the intestines of virtually any vertebrate, hence we have *Giardia muris* in rodents, *Giardia agilis* in amphibians, *Giardia psittaci* and *Giardia ardeae* in birds, and *Giardia microti* in voles and muskrats,[6] but *Giardia lamblia* is the only species that affects humans, mopping up our nutrients and triggering painful cramps. These abdominal cramps are a sign that our digestive system is under attack, but Giardia is a disturbingly crafty little microbe. It can change the proteins on its surface, and doing this allows it to pass unrecognised and unvanquished through the gut, often managing to linger for many years because the antibodies produced to seek out and destroy it are unable to recognise it in its new guise. By the time new antibodies have been developed, the Giardia will have changed its appearance yet again.

Once it finds a suitable home where the host's immune system is compromised, can no longer resist and has virtually given up the fight, the Giardia will begin to colonise and establish itself, feeding and breeding so the species can continue. It is not in the parasite's interest to kill off the host as that would be counterproductive; its very existence depends on the continual supply of nourishment being provided daily, and the longer it remains undetected, the better it is for Giardia and its offspring.

This coexistence can last for many years. During this time, the host will suffer a collection of seemingly unrelated symptoms which will confuse the medical professionals trying to help them; the Giardia will be happily living a strong and productive life inhabiting various parts of the host's body. Many of those providing this safe haven for Giardia will learn to live with the digestive disruptions and other health issues it causes, and may even have been given a label to explain their chronic condition.

Giardia relies on its host retaining a reasonable level of health in order for it to survive, but sometimes its presence will severely weaken the host and disease eventually takes over, destroying the parasite's habitat. However, a majority of infected people, remain well enough to tolerate the discomfort of an infestation, thus allowing the undiscovered and untreated parasite to rapidly colonise the entire intestinal tract.[7] It takes just 14 to 16 hours for it to produce infective cysts that are excreted through the host's faeces.[8] These are capable of surviving outside the body for weeks or months, ready to be picked up by anyone who unwittingly takes in water or food that has been contaminated with them.

Swallowing and ingesting just 10 of these cysts is enough to cause giardiasis. Depending on factors such as the strength of a person's immune system and age (children and the elderly are more susceptible), an infection with Giardia can result in a sufferer becoming an asymptomatic carrier (if they are lucky), or developing a wide range of unexplained symptoms. The most obvious of these is the chronic diarrhoea mentioned above, along with its repercussions, such as severe malabsorption of nutrients, which affects around 200 million people a year worldwide. But Giardia can also trigger other health issues and, when diarrhoea is not a symptom, and for many people it is not, it can be hard to get a diagnosis.

Recognising symptoms

Digestive problems

Although it takes about five to seven days for Giardia to colonise the entire intestinal tract, it can take just 24 hours for the whole digestive system to be thrown into turmoil. It is not unusual for a person to go from one day being perfectly healthy, with a bowel that is functioning normally, to the next day being severely bloated with wind, nausea and diarrhoea, or constipation, or all of the above. As more time passes, and the infection takes hold, a sufferer can change from being an outgoing, happy-go-lucky person, full of confidence, to being an unhappy introvert beset with insecurities and fears that make them unrecognisable from the character they once were. Even within a very short space of time, their energy levels are likely to fall dramatically. Coping with long-term diarrhoea is debilitating, stressful and potentially isolating. Soon the sufferer is caught in a spiral of health problems, which causes their stress levels to rise, with all the additional repercussions that that situation brings.

If diarrhoea is the main problem, just trying to leave the house for work each day can become a challenge. Functioning on a daily basis can become a nightmare and many of my patients just want to hibernate. They become withdrawn and seem frail and preoccupied – nothing like the strong and healthy people they were before Giardia entered their lives.

Increased allergic problems

Asthma, hay fever and other allergic conditions may suddenly appear, often having even more impact than the digestive issues. This is because the malabsorption of essential nutrients and a disturbed gut flora, caused by the parasite's activity, are weakening the immune system's ability to deal with these conditions. The parasite also produces antigens, which impair the body's natural ability to protect itself. When Giardia is the root cause of these allergic problems, the symptoms should disappear as soon as the parasite has been killed off.

Sleep problems

Sleeplessness is another problem I frequently see in people with a Giardia infestation. This is because parasites are often more active at night, and Giardia is no exception. It is not unusual to be woken in the night by sweating, diarrhoea, itching and a feeling of 'things' crawling under the skin as it busily feeds, breeds and excretes its waste through its plasma membrane, as Laura describes.

Laura's story

Last year, having returned from a lovely holiday in Norfolk with my family, I started to experience a strange feeling when I was lying in bed preparing for sleep. I had a weird sensation of something bubbling and gathering in my gut. It seemed to be building in strength, with an intention of pushing up through my gullet and exploding in my chest. It was really frightening, and when it first happened I thought I was going to have a heart attack. It only happened at night, and only when I was lying down.

Not wishing to be too dramatic, but very worried, I went to my GP. It had occurred to me it could be the start of an aortic aneurysm, and I also knew it was important to seek early treatment if that was the case. My GP was great; he couldn't find anything obvious to explain the symptoms I was getting, and sent me off to the hospital for an ultrasound scan on my belly. Thankfully it was totally clear and everything appeared to be working perfectly normally.

The problem continued though, and with no other symptoms than this sensation of 'whooshing' and imminent explosion in my chest, I visited the Willow Herbal Centre and met Sue Koten.

> Through a process of questions and testing, Sue diagnosed a Giardia infestation in my gut. I was amazed – I'd never heard of Giardia or the havoc it can cause if left untreated.
>
> Sue gave me a herbal spray containing wormwood to use for five days and I am very happy to say, it solved the problem. Amazing!

Skin problems

As well as the digestive problems associated with a Giardia infestation, a patient might also experience a breakout of small spots, itchy skin, or hot, raised blotchy patches known as urticaria (nettle rash). This is an inflammatory immune response and it is my belief, based on experience with my patients, that if a person has giardiasis, then any inflammatory response is exacerbated.

Food intolerance

Eating can also become an issue as foods previously eaten with impunity now start to create problems, becoming indigestible and causing wind, griping pains, diarrhoea and nausea. About 50% of my patients become gluten-intolerant when suffering from giardiasis (see Chapter 4, page 34). This is because the parasite has caused the microvilli (microscopic projections that vastly increase the internal surface area of the gut) lining the small intestine to shorten, and therefore some foods are not absorbed efficiently. Cutting culprit foods out of the diet helps some people and can make life more manageable. However, this does not address the underlying problem of the parasite. Patients, unaware they have giardiasis, often stop eating fresh fruit and vegetables because these shoot straight through the body, but doing this will cause sufferers to miss out on the many valuable nutrients these foods provide and will further weaken an already compromised digestive system.

Basically, when a person is infected with Giardia, they are sharing their body with a vast and constantly growing family of uninvited guests, and the results can be debilitating, devastating and, if left untreated, life changing.

The lifecycle of Giardia

Giardia is a parasitic amoeba, a single-celled organism of the type known as a 'protozoon' (plural, 'protozoa'). It has a two-stage lifecycle consisting of the trophozoite (stage one), which is the feeding stage, and the cyst (stage two), which is the infective stage.

Stage 1 – Trophozoite (feeding) stage

The 'trophozoite' is the actively dividing stage of the parasite. From its tiny (12 x 6 microns) pear-shaped body (one micron is about a fifth of the size of a red blood cell), protrude four pairs of 'flagella' – wavy lash-like 'legs' that enable it to travel inside the body. A ventral disc, with its suction cup having a snail-like appearance, is made up of microtubules, allowing it to attach itself to the intestines where it will feed on the victim's nutrients.

These trophozoites emerge from the cysts that have been inadvertently swallowed. The acidic environment of the stomach causes the cysts to rupture and, with the help of its flagella to push its way through the cyst wall, the trophozoite emerges into the more alkaline duodenum (the section of the gut after the stomach).

This brand new protozoon that emerges from the ruptured cyst then undergoes transformation, resulting in two new trophozoites. It is these new trophozoites that are the cause of giardiasis, and the start of the digestive problems.

With the trophozoites doubling in number every six to eight hours, the digestive tract can soon become overrun with them, giving its lining (mucosa) the appearance of a cobblestone beach. Each cobblestone is a trophozoite busily feeding off glucose, attaching itself to the mucosa of the duodenum and jejunum by its ventral disc; this suction pad anchors it securely while it starts its feeding frenzy, gorging on nutrients that should have been absorbed by the host's body.

By now, the host will have started to experience feelings of being unwell, as symptoms of fatigue and digestive disorder take over, giving a clear marker that the body has been invaded.

Because of the suction action of the disc of the trophozoite, the parasite is not swept away with digested food but can stay feeding, fulfilling its requirements. It can also detach itself, move to a different feeding ground, and reattach as cells are naturally shed off the lining of the intestinal tract.

Giardia are killed off if medication is taken (herbs or antimicrobials) that prevent it from attaching to the epithelial cells (the cells that line the gut and form the mucosa). This is because when the parasite cannot feed it dies off and is passed out in the faeces.

If the host has a strong immune system it should also start attacking the Giardia. However, Giardia has learned to adapt to its surroundings and survive very effectively and efficiently. It is capable of changing its appearance by altering the proteins on its surface membrane, as I have mentioned, to disguise itself so that the host's immune system is unable to recognise it, thereby leaving the trophozoites to continue feeding and breeding for years.

A person who has been previously infected should have antibodies that recognise the parasite and can kill it off, but it is when the body's defence system starts attacking the Giardia that it begins the process of altering its appearance, which is why it can remain undetected for long periods of time.

Untreated, the Giardia trophozoites can also reach and invade the gallbladder, which is connected to the duodenum via the common bile duct (see Chapter 8, page 74), and the pancreas, which is connected to this first part of the small intestine via the pancreatic duct (see Chapter 9, page 82), causing the organs to malfunction, with repercussions that can include interference with insulin production in the pancreas.

Giardia depend on bile, which is produced by the liver and delivered via the gallbladder, to go into their cyst stage, so they tend to congregate around the entrance of the bile duct. They may also localise in the biliary tract to avoid the relative acidity of the duodenum. The mean diameter of the human common bile duct is 4.1 mm, but this can vary to as much as 11 mm in patients with gallstones.[9] This means Giardia, which measure about 12 x 6 microns, as previously mentioned, are capable of entering the gallbladder via the common bile duct.

Giardia can live in a slightly acidic environment of pH 6.38–7.02 (pH 7 is neutral – neither acid nor alkaline), which the duodenum and upper jejunum supply. It is here that the Giardia trophozoites attach themselves and feed by absorption constantly.

Stage 2 – The cyst stage

One microgram of stool may contain as many as 300 million cysts.[10] Each one is an oval-shaped resistant structure with a very thick protein wall that enables it to survive the harsh conditions outside a host's body. Infection then starts when a potential host picks up cysts from the parasite.

Giardia in its cyst form is robust enough to resist environmental destruction and disinfection and, because of this extraordinary resilience, cysts can be picked up from contaminated water, or any surface that has come into contact with human or animal faeces and has not been adequately cleaned. According to the Centers for Disease Control (CDC) in the US, it takes three to four cups of bleach per gallon of water to kill off Giardia. The cysts are also almost completely immune to the effects of chlorine.

Travellers, beware!

As the WHO figures indicate, Giardia infection is high around the globe and care should always be taken with hygiene when travelling abroad. However, it seems antimalarial treatment can keep Giardia at bay. Both giardiasis and malaria are caused by protozoan infestations and can give symptoms of headache, sweating, nausea, vomiting, chills and diarrhoea.

I have noticed that some of my patients who have taken antimalarial tablets while travelling seem to have had symptoms suggestive of giardiasis prior to going abroad, but were symptom-free until they stopped taking the antimalarial medication, usually when they got back home to the UK. It seems the antimalarials have kept their symptoms under control but without actually eliminating the parasite, as this next story illustrates.

Celia's story

My patient, Celia, had been ill for years but then started taking Lariam (mefloquine) two weeks before travelling to Kenya, and was surprised to find she was perfectly well for the entire five months that she spent there. She continued with the drug for two weeks after returning home, but a week after stopping the medication she became ill with vomiting and diarrhoea, and after three months of constant problems, her GP diagnosed giardiasis. She was prescribed a four-day course of the antibiotic metronidazole. This halted the severity of her symptoms, but she continued to suffer from daily bloating and cramps, frequent episodes of constipation and cycles of random vomiting or offensive-smelling diarrhoea (for more information on the malaria connection, see Chapter 11, page 109).

I treated Celia with wormwood for the giardiasis, along with herbs to support and treat her kidneys and gallbladder, as I had also detected problems with these. She was sensitive to gluten, so I recommended she eliminate that from her diet, and within a week she was much better.

Chapter 1

In the chapters that follow I will explain how to prevent Giardia infection, and when to suspect it could be the real cause of other health problems that may be present. However, I would like to end this chapter with the experience of another of my patients, who I will call 'Julia'.

Julia's story

It all started with my black labrador, Daisy, becoming horribly ill with diarrhoea that eventually had to be treated with the antibiotic metronidazole. Soon afterwards, I also became ill with stomach cramps and diarrhoea, and I still had an upset stomach three weeks later. By this time even liquid vitamins and probiotic powders were causing me to suffer griping stomach pains.

My mood and energy levels fluctuated wildly. I was restless at night, agitated and nauseous. My stools were pale and orange in colour, greasy and horribly smelly. However, when my doctor tested a sample, nothing showed up, and I was told to go away and get on with my life.

This should have been reassuring, but I was continuing to get a lot of diarrhoea, and now I had frequent headaches too, so I asked my GP for a private referral to a consultant gastroenterologist. The consultant listened to my story, said it sounded like Giardia lamblia and gave me a prescription for metronidazole 400 mg.

I took the drugs, but three weeks later I still felt fatigued and unable to make the shortest trip to the shops without returning exhausted. I had a metallic taste in my mouth and had lost 10 pounds (4.5 kilos) in weight. By this time, I'd had to cancel numerous activities – birthday parties and a wedding. Where had my nice, normal life gone?

It was only when I found Susan Koten and started treatment with her that things began to improve. Susan was convinced I still had the parasite and prescribed wormwood, together with a herbal remedy for my kidneys and gallbladder as I had discomfort in my right kidney and sensitivity in my small intestines.

Five days later, I exploded with emotion and I knew I was better. Ten days after starting treatment, when I saw Susan again, she confirmed, by testing with kinesiology, I was now clear of the parasite.

The very next day I went on holiday to Venice and was able to drink beer and wine, and eat salads and masses of gelato, forgetting all about parasites.

I felt fine, remembering too late what Susan had told me – that the parasite loves sweet foods and that I should stick with cooked vegetables and avoid salads while I was away. Back home, I woke with a start knowing that the giardiasis was back. I was vomiting and retching violently while simultaneously passing watery diarrhoea. I was bringing up lots of green bile, burping and suffering headaches and a rapid heart beat.

Susan put me back on wormwood, and this time it took 10 days to clear the parasite – but that was a small price to pay after the five months of misery I had endured before discovering this herbal cure.

Julia did contract giardiasis again as she says, and took herbs which cleared her condition, but Giardia is a very common parasite and unless the immune system is strengthened and the body's environment is made less inviting for Giardia to live in, we remain at risk of contracting it again and must take more precautions to avoid infection in the first place. For this see Chapter 9 on prevention.

Summary

Giardia, a microscopic intestinal parasite, has been known about for a long time but is usually associated with foreign travel and third-world communities. This has meant its prevalence in the UK has largely gone unnoticed by the medical community and has seen the range of symptoms associated with infestation, frequently misdiagnosed. Both animals and humans can be infected and this protozoan parasite is using our bodies as a breeding and feeding ground weakening its host, while thriving and flourishing undetected.

Many people hosting this parasite have been diagnosed as suffering from irritable bowel syndrome (IBS) and in Chapter 2 we look at the various options available to health professionals for finding and identifying this uninvited guest. We also discuss the similarities between a Giardia infestation and the IBS diagnosis – as my evidence suggests, in many cases, the ignorance around Giardia and its presence in the UK may have led to the parasite being missed as a cause of this debilitating and costly complaint.

Chapter 2

Getting a diagnosis

As previously mentioned, there were 4492 confirmed cases of giardiasis in England and Wales in 2016.[1] This translates into less than 0.1% of the population but, from my own experience of diagnosing Giardia infestations and treating patients, I suspect the actual number is far higher.

An article published in the *British Medical Journal* (*BMJ*) in October 2016 says the incidence of giardiasis is underestimated in the United Kingdom 'because of the lack of diagnostic sensitivity of traditional faecal microscopy' and also because of the mistaken belief it is mostly contracted by people who travel abroad.[2] This is supported by Government figures showing only 7% of the reported cases of giardiasis in England, Wales and Northern Ireland, are associated with foreign travel.

Many of the patients I see, who are infected with Giardia, have not been abroad prior to the infection, but generally doctors only test for parasites in patients who have unexplained gastric and bowel disorders if they have recently spent time overseas.

In my experience, giardiasis can cause a number of health problems for years – often mistaken for irritable bowel syndrome (IBS as it is commonly known) – going untested, undiagnosed and untreated. In my practice, I often see patients suffering from IBS, and time and time again I find Giardia present in their system. When I administer my herbal remedy for parasites, the symptoms clear up, often within days. A quote from Rachel's story is a clear example.

> **Rachel's story**
>
> *After suffering many years with IBS symptoms and going to countless doctors and trying endless complementary therapies, I finally found what I believe to be the root cause – parasites. It is with Susan Koten's help that I have been able to eradicate them and in the process rid myself of all IBS symptoms. I spent years seeing one specialist after another and none of them even hinted to me that parasites could be the cause. Since using her herbal parasite tincture I have eradicated my Giardia infection.*

IBS is the term used for a collection of unrelated symptoms which are debilitating, and sometimes life changing, for those unfortunate enough to have the problem. Since there is no known cause for IBS, there is no known cure, and people with this diagnosis are destined to live a life of unpredictable illness, special diets, bouts of pain, sudden dashes to the nearest toilet facility and all the other symptoms related to a dysfunctional digestive system.

Testing for Giardia

Conventional diagnosis of giardiasis is based on the results of three stool tests over a period of days. The results may also be confirmed by the more sensitive 'enzyme-linked immunosorbent assay' (ELISA) test. This tests for the Giardia antigens in a patient's stool sample to determine if the parasite is present. Occasionally a String Test (see below) might also be offered. Private clinics additionally offer a comprehensive parasitology stool test, to look for infestations, while alternative practitioners use various options for diagnosing the problem. Applied kinesiology (muscle testing) is a reliable diagnostic tool and the one I use in my practice.

Stool ova and parasite (O&P) tests

Patients are asked to provide samples from three consecutive stools because Giardia is notoriously hard to detect from a single sample. The cysts are shed intermittently, so one sample may be clear while the next may contain them.

Three stool examinations have been shown to have a 90% success rate in identifying Giardia, compared with 50-70% when only a single sample is examined.[3] However, even with three stool tests, a negative result does not mean the patient is not infected with Giardia.

ELISA stool test

If the ova and parasite tests have proved negative, but the doctor still suspects giardiasis, the patient may be offered a stool antigen enzyme linked immunosorbent assay (ELISA) test, as mentioned above. This test is designed to pick up evidence of the *Giardia lamblia*-specific antigen and is more sensitive in detecting its presence than the ova and parasite test.

String test

If the ELISA test has also failed to identify Giardia yet the parasite is still suspected, the patient could be offered the String test. This involves swallowing a gelatine capsule attached to a length of nylon string. Over a period of a few hours, the capsule gathers samples from the patient's intestine and stomach. It is then pulled back out through the mouth and sent to a laboratory for analysis.

Comprehensive parasitology stool test

The comprehensive parasitology stool test is a combination of the O&P and ELISA tests which not only examines a patient's stool sample for evidence of parasitic infestation, but also uses the powerful microscope technology to identifiy moulds, yeasts, bacterial overgrowth, pH imbalance and much more. It is a fast and accurate method of detection to identify what is inside the gut.

Testing for irritable bowel syndrome (IBS)

In all my years of treating patients who believe they have IBS, I have formed my own views of the condition and they do not tally with conventional thoughts about it, but first let us look at what these conventional views are.

IBS is listed as a chronic condition and affects one in five of the population of England and Wales, according to 'Patient Info', a British-based internet service providing information for healthcare practitioners and patients.[4] That is 20% of the population, or around 14 million people, and although anybody of any age can be affected, it usually begins to manifest in early adulthood, and then continues throughout the life of the sufferer.

The most commonly listed symptoms of IBS are:
• abdominal pain
• bloating
• a change in bowel habit, such as a change in elimination frequency or the onset of diarrhoea and/or constipation.

Obtaining a diagnosis can take a long time, sometimes years, as the symptoms change and patients develop coping strategies that help them manage the problems and stops them seeking help. Many sufferers do not revisit their doctor after the initial consultation if nothing abnormal is found, but continue to live with the problem and get on with their lives as best they can. Without a causal factor or 'bio-marker' to confirm IBS, clinicians follow a standard protocol which involves discussing the patient's symptoms and the frequency of occurrence, taking a full medical history, and also conducting a physical examination. If any 'red flags' are indicated during this consultation, such as rectal bleeding, or unexplained weight loss, the doctor will order various blood and stool tests to eliminate other bowel or digestive disorders, but eventually, if none are found, the patient will be told they have IBS.

It is my belief that the Giardia parasite is more widespread than so far reported and that a large proportion of IBS sufferers are actually Giardia carriers.

Testing for inflammatory bowel disease (IBD)

The symptoms for IBS are only slightly different from the most commonly listed symptoms of IBD, which is the umbrella term for inflammatory conditions such as Crohn's disease, which can affect any part of the bowel as well as the mouth, and ulcerative colitis, which affects the colon only. They are:

- abdominal pain
- swelling or cramping
- recurring or bloody diarrhoea
- weight loss
- extreme tiredness.

A change in bowel habit, such as the onset of loose, more frequent stools, is also one of the three main symptoms of bowel cancer. The others are blood in the stools and abdominal pain, making these 'red flags'.

There is a lot of overlap in these symptoms. Although patients diagnosed with IBS, IBD or bowel cancer typically present with abdominal pain and a change in bowel habit, these same symptoms can occur with giardiasis.

If a patient's symptoms hint at possible IBD, which, according to Crohn's & Colitis UK (a web-based support network) affects more than 300,000 people in the UK, a series of tests is available to confirm the diagnosis. These range from blood and stool analysis to endoscopies, ultrasounds, MRI scans and X-rays. Doctors are looking for signs of inflammation. The presence of faecal calprotectin, a substance released into the intestine in response to inflammation, can distinguish IBD from IBS. However, the inflammation may still need to be confirmed with a further procedure, such as an endoscopy (a test which enables doctors to inspect the bowel using a flexible tube inserted through the anus or mouth, an X-ray (often using a barium meal which coats the lining of the gut to give a clearer image), an ultrasound or a magnetic resonance imaging (MRI) scan. Ultrasound is useful for picking up areas of accumulated fluid, and thickened, inflamed parts of the bowel. MRI comes into its own in detecting abscesses and fistulas (abnormal tunnels in the bowel).

Manual muscle testing

Despite all of these powerful diagnostic tools, many people still present themselves to me with gut problems. Some arrive having already been diagnosed with giardiasis, either via their general practitioner or by private testing using the comprehensive parasitology stool test. Others come because the tests have failed to find the parasite, and all other causes for their problems have been excluded. I use muscle testing to confirm or rule out a diagnosis of giardiasis and to detect any other underlying causes of their digestive problems. This form of testing is not offered by a conventional doctor or at a conventional clinic. However, it is a method I routinely use in the diagnostic process with all my patients.

Manual muscle testing (MMT), also known as applied kinesiology (AK), involves no blood, stool, or any other human substance. There is no need for laboratory testing, or even medical equipment. This is a diagnostic method that simply involves the patient holding out his or her arm while the practitioner applies gentle pressure to the arm and silently poses a number of questions.

I learned how to muscle test for Giardia and other organisms while studying under the British Institute for Allergy and Environmental Therapy. I became a member in December 1997 and have been using this method successfully and accurately (judging by results) ever since. The Institute was formed in January 1987 to bring together a group of allergy practitioners, all of whom had undergone the same course of instruction and who practise allergy therapy in a similar way, using muscle testing as a means of diagnosis. There are currently over 300 therapists on the Institute's register, which is available to the general public who are seeking treatment (www.kinesiologyfederation.co.uk). Membership is open only to those people who have satisfactorily completed the Institute's training.

With over 1200 muscle tests to choose from, I am able to detect a wide range of pathogens and environmental issues, quickly identifying which organs are affected and getting a clearer understanding of what is causing the imbalance in health, so I can prescribe the appropriate herbs to treat each individual. Giardia may not be the only parasite invading the body; it could be only one part of the problem.

Applied kinesiology (AK) was developed by Michigan chiropractor George J Goodheart, Jr, and is now used by many complementary health practitioners. Dr Goodheart discovered that the strength or weakness of every muscle was connected to the health, or lack of health, of a specific corresponding organ, and that positive physical stimuli, like vitamin supplements, would increase the strength of the muscles that he tested. He also saw that negative stimuli would cause those muscles to become weak. To him, this implied that, at a deep level, the body knows what is 'good' for it and what is not.

Clinical kinesiology (CK) developed out of applied kinesiology. In 1968, Dr Alan Beardall, who had just graduated as a chiropractor, became one of Dr Goodheart's students. Dr Beardall went on to develop over 250 specific muscle tests to diagnose and evaluate structural, chemical and mental aspects of health. He also discovered a way of communicating with the patient's subconscious which enabled the body to reveal underlying causes of health problems.

I have been studying and treating patients affected by Giardia for over 20 years and muscle testing has allowed me to get a clearer understanding of its presence in the body and help in determining the correct treatment protocol.

When I use muscle testing to diagnose a problem I am tapping into the patient's subconscious, which knows precisely what the body needs to rebuild itself. I am looking for the energetic strength of each organ that I am testing. Muscle testing enables me to identify whether there is a viral, parasitic, fungal or bacterial problem. I can also be more accurate in advising on what foods to eat and which to avoid, and whether there is a gluten sensitivity, as there is in many Giardia patients. This form of testing gives me a great advantage over conventional methods as it is non-invasive and can be performed in my therapy room at the start of the consultation.

It is useful to note the body's main purpose is survival, and it will do everything possible to continue this process. Just observe the growth of a new baby in the womb. We do not consciously have to get involved in its development once a pregnancy has been established, but just be guided and allow this creation to take place. Everything our body does is for survival unless we consciously or subconsciously decide to hinder this process by putting up barriers and blocks so the life force energy cannot flow freely. Muscle testing allows the examiner to tap into the body's innate wisdom and determine what is beneficial to its health and what will hinder its wellbeing. We can be very detached from our physical bodies and are too often preoccupied by false concepts of what we really need.

Here's a crude example: we may believe that we need to get blind drunk to have a good time, and that unless we are sick at the end of it, this good time has not been achieved. But in fact, the body, which is trying to stay well, disgorges the alcohol in an attempt to stop itself from being poisoned. If we tapped into our body's inner, subconscious wisdom, it would tell us it does not want excess alcohol in the first place. Muscle testing is a way of accessing this inner, subconscious wisdom. It gives us a very good insight into what the body really wants.

Typically, if left untreated, Giardia can create years of digestive problems, as my patient Sophie's story illustrates even though she underwent conventional testing methods to try to get a diagnosis.

Sophie's story

Everyone expects their fair share of tummy upsets when they go on holiday to Asia and the Far East; it's part of the package. But, when I went off back-packing soon after leaving university, I seemed to fare incredibly well. For nearly a year, I had the bare minimum of problems. It was only when I reached Cambodia that my luck finally ran out, as my arrival coincided with the most catastrophic floods the country had seen in generations. Streets that had days earlier been full of cars were now rivers with boats ferrying bewildered locals and tourists.

Ground water was silently rising around us, and one morning I woke in my hostel to find my back-pack floating next to me. The sewerage systems had burst and my friends and I had to wade through knee-deep filth.

That's when the dreaded traveller's tummy finally struck with a vengeance. I had very severe diarrhoea and I was vomiting, producing foul-smelling wind.

My first thought was that I needed to be somewhere I could get myself sorted out. So, with zero energy, I pushed myself to get to Bangkok, for medical help. A series of tests finally revealed I was infected with worms and something called Giardia.

I didn't know what that was, but I was told that an antibiotic would clear it up and, indeed, I was much better when I was discharged, and able to continue with my gap year.

But, moving on into New Zealand and Australia, my tummy was never quite the same again. It seemed to react to all sorts of foods, and I became obsessed with trying to work out exactly what my triggers were. My symptoms were nothing like as bad as they'd been back in Bangkok so that mystery diagnosis of Giardia was no longer on my radar, but, back home in the UK, I was still suffering from loose bowels and foul wind, and I felt embarrassed and very unladylike.

My GP thought it was just IBS, but I could not accept that, and eventually managed to get a referral to the London Hospital for Tropical Diseases. However, even there, I sailed through a barrage of tests with no satisfactory diagnosis. It seemed that I, like so many millions with debilitating IBS, was just expected to accept my situation and get on with it.

Over the years that followed this became harder and harder for me to do. As I trained, and then worked, as an architect, I worried about meetings, office toilets, meals out. And, socially, I hated always having to consider the content of everything I was offered.

Somewhere along the line I noticed that eating spicy food had fairly disastrous effects on my bowels so I started avoiding that. Then I paid to see a nutritionist, who recommended also cutting out sugar and lactose. I did all this, but nothing seemed to change. I even tried colonic irrigation and was informed by the therapist that I had a lot of gas in my gut. That much I already knew!

Years carried on rolling by until, with a particularly bad attack, I decided to revive my attempts at sorting myself out. This time my Google search threw up a newspaper article about a medical herbalist called Susan Koten who specialised in the treatment of Giardia. The word leaped off the screen at me, taking me back to my early 20s and that diagnosis in Bangkok. Testimonials praised Susan for having cured patients after years of symptoms that sounded just like mine – and I knew I had to see her.

Her method of diagnosis, using muscle testing, is hard for many to get their heads around, but I'd already experienced this with a nutritionist and I wasn't fazed. It took Susan just minutes to work out that I still had Giardia in my system. She explained that it is a microscopic parasite that rapidly reproduces in the body, causing stomach cramps, nausea and digestive problems.

The antibiotics I'd been given all those years ago in Bangkok should have killed off the Giardia. However, if they had failed to do so completely, the parasites could have reproduced again. I left Susan's practice with a tonic containing wormwood – also known as Artemisia annua. It sounds amazing, I know, but within 10 days, I had 'normal' bowels again. What's more, I could eat what I liked, even spicy food, without worrying. My course of treatment had lasted just seven days.

I was shocked that I'd suffered unnecessarily for so long and that Giardia was so poorly understood and treated by the medical profession.

Summary

Given the low incidence of recorded Giardia infestations in England and Wales, the high incidence of recorded cases of IBS, and the similarity of symptoms for both complaints, it is not unreasonable to conclude there is more to be done before a patient is given the uncertainty of an IBS diagnosis.

Educating health practitioners about the prevalence of Giardia in the UK and ensuring they routinely test for Giardia using the ELISA test would, in my view, capture many hitherto undetected cases of giardiasis and save patients and the health service many years of uncertainty and cost.

Educating ourselves, as well, about this parasite, and being aware of its existence in our community, will enable us both to lower the risk of infection and to seek help should we become infected. In Chapter 3 we will discuss what to look for and how to get help if we suspect its presence.

Chapter 3

Checking for Giardia

As previously mentioned, giardiasis (infection with Giardia) can sometimes be present but with no gastric symptoms at all, in which case it becomes particularly difficult to get a conventional diagnosis. In my experience, however, all the following, listed in alphabetical order, can be linked to infection with this parasite and are good reasons to consider being tested for its presence in the body:

- **Allergies and asthma:** Studies have shown a distinct correlation between giardiasis and allergy, possibly because the infection damages the mucous membrane of the intestine and this increases antigen activity and sensitisation towards food antigens.[1] A Venezuelan study found that children were significantly more likely to suffer from asthma-like wheezing if they had a protozoan infection such as giardiasis.[2]

- **Apathy:** A feeling of withdrawal from the world is common as sufferers try to cope with the symptoms of giardiasis and the loss of energy that they feel as a result.

- **B12 deficiency:** Because of the impact of Giardia infestation on absorption of nutrients, it can lead to a vitamin B12 deficiency, resulting in a wide range of symptoms from fatigue and depression to muscular problems that may even be mistaken for multiple sclerosis.

- **Bad breath:** This is caused by an inefficient breakdown of foods, creating fermentation that surfaces through the mouth.
- **Bloating:** This is caused by gases created by the fermentation of foods that have not been properly broken down.
- **Chills and fever:** The body's temperature will rise, to try to kill off the parasite, and then fall again, creating chills and a mild fever. This is the body's natural defence against infection.
- **Chronic cough:** If the cause of a long-term cough is proving hard to diagnose, then parasites should be considered as a possible cause, especially if there are bowel and/or digestive issues accompanying it.
- **Chronic fatigue syndrome:** Loss of energy is another result of nutrient depletion, caused by giardiasis. A Norwegian study of 53 people with chronic fatigue diagnosed Giardia as the underlying cause in over 50% of participants. All had contracted the parasite five years earlier in a waterborne outbreak of giardiasis in 2004 in Bergen, Norway, which had affected around 5000 people.[3]
- **Coeliac disease:** This is an autoimmune disorder, causing the immune system to attack the body in the presence of gluten, but its symptoms can also be mimicked by giardiasis (see Chapter 4, page 35).
- **Constipation:** Having bowel movements less than three times per week, with stools that are hard, small and difficult to expel, counts as constipation, and Giardia can cause this by interfering with the transition and movement of waste through the intestinal tract and making the colon muscles sluggish.

- **Depression:** In my experience there is often a feeling of hopelessness and disillusionment in trying to come to terms with an undiagnosed Giardia infestation and its symptoms.
- **Diabetes:** When Giardia gets into the pancreas it can interfere with patients' insulin levels (see Chapter 9, page 82).
- **Diarrhoea:** This can become chronic if giardiasis goes untreated, and it is not unknown for it to continue for years. Frequent bouts of diarrhoea every day can cause severe potassium loss as a result and this can lead to muscle weakness (see below). Research has found that taking zinc supplements can reduce the rate of diarrhoea caused by giardiasis.[4]
- **Distended abdomen:** Undigested foods ferment and cause gas, which bloats the stomach.
- **Eye problems:** Damage to the cells of the retina can lead to lesions on the eyes.[5] The link with Giardia is still not fully understood.
- **Food intolerances:** Giardia infestation causes inflammation and damage to the intestinal wall, creating a leaky gut and food intolerances, such as of gluten. For more about this, see Chapter 4 (page 34).
- **Growth retardation:** Failure to thrive and stunted growth in children are also linked to giardiasis,[6] as the parasites can interfere with the uptake of nutrients.
- **Headaches:** In my experience, many patients have headaches that can clear up when Giardia is eliminated. Christopher's case in Chapter 10 is a good example of this.
- **Irritable bowel syndrome (IBS):** Following the 2004 Bergen outbreak, researchers linked *Giardia duodenalis* infections to post-infectious IBS.[7]
- **Lethargy:** This is often linked to a gluten intolerance,

one of the repercussions of Giardia infestation.

- **Mucus in stools:** Especially if the mucus has a jelly-like appearance, it could be carrying the trophozoites and cysts that are being excreted.
- **Muscle/joint pain:** Giardia infections can trigger reactive arthritis or synovitis by altering the body's defence against infections. Reactive arthritis can cause pain and swelling in the knees, ankles, heels, toes and fingers, and constant low back pain, which can be worse at night or in the morning. Inflammatory arthritis has also been linked with Giardia infestations, and can be the cause of painful knees and ankles.[8]
- **Nausea:** This is caused by foods that the infested gut is unable to digest properly and an associated undiagnosed gluten intolerance.
- **Noisy intestines:** These are caused by poorly digested foods fermenting and creating gases that produce gurgling sounds.
- **Offensive-smelling stools:** This is caused by the putrefaction of foods that cannot be properly digested.
- **Shortness of breath:** This is a symptom of Giardia creating an allergic asthmatic response.
- **Skin problems:** Urticaria (nettle rash) has been associated with a Giardia infestation.[9]
- **Sleep disturbance:** Giardia can become more active at night and may interfere with sleep patterns.
- **Stomach cramps:** This may be due to the inability to digest foods (especially gluten) efficiently, which will create gas and wind, creating cramps.
- **Sweating:** Giardia may induce a low-grade fever, which can give rise to sweating.
- **Tooth grinding (bruxism):** This is the abnormal unconscious grinding, clenching and gnashing of the teeth, especially at night. I have noticed that when teeth

grinders infected with Giardia are treated, they stop grinding their teeth.

- **Vomiting:** This is caused by high levels of toxins given off by Giardia and foods not being digested effectively. Nausea is more common than actually vomiting with Giardia.
- **Weakness:** This is a result of being undernourished because of foods not being absorbed efficiently.
- **Weight loss:** This is caused by malnourishment due to inefficient digestion and / or a restricted diet.
- **Wind:** This is due to undigested foods fermenting and giving off gases.
- **Yellow/cream-coloured stools:** This is a sign that the gallbladder has become infected and bile salts are unable to travel from the liver into the gut via the gallbladder and bile duct.

When new patients come to my clinic I ask them to check the list below and tick which of the symptoms (as mentioned above) apply to them. The more they tick, the more likely it is that Giardia is present in their system and they need to be tested. The symptoms listed are drawn from my many years of treating patients with Giardia infestation. Indeed, one of my patients had over 20 symptoms, ranging from gastric disturbances and nausea to joint and muscle pain, chronic fatigue, depression and memory problems.

For anyone suspecting they may unwittingly be providing a safe haven for this prolific little parasite, completing this health check could prove useful in helping to confirm its presence.

Health checklist

- ☐ Allergies
- ☐ Apathy
- ☐ Asthma
- ☐ B12 deficiency
- ☐ Bad breath
- ☐ Bloating
- ☐ Burping
- ☐ Chills
- ☐ Chronic fatigue
- ☐ Coeliac disease
- ☐ Constipation
- ☐ Depression
- ☐ Diabetes
- ☐ Diarrhoea
- ☐ Distended abdomen
- ☐ Ear, nose and throat problems
- ☐ Food intolerances
- ☐ Headaches
- ☐ IBD (inflammatory bowel disease)
- ☐ IBS (irritable bowel syndrome)
- ☐ Inability to concentrate
- ☐ Joint pain
- ☐ Lethargy
- ☐ Memory deficits
- ☐ Mucus in stools
- ☐ Muscle pain
- ☐ Nausea
- ☐ Noisy intestines
- ☐ Offensive-smelling stools
- ☐ Chronic cough
- ☐ Shortness of breath
- ☐ Skin problems
- ☐ Sleep disturbance
- ☐ Stomach cramps
- ☐ Sweating
- ☐ Teeth grinding
- ☐ Vomiting
- ☐ Weakness
- ☐ Weight loss
- ☐ Wind
- ☐ Yellow/cream-coloured stools

Getting help

For those who suspect Giardia may be present in their system, there are several options available for confirming it.

a) Visit the GP and request an ELISA stool test to confirm if Giardia is present.

b) Pay for a comprehensive parasitology stool test (see page 16) to confirm a Giardia infestation and take the result to your GP or qualified medical practitioner.

As I have said, an undetected Giardia infestation can be debilitating and frightening as it gradually erodes a sufferer's general state of health and wellbeing.

Sally's story

Having had blood tests return all-clear and doctors showing no further interest, I visited Susan, who concluded from her examination that I had a parasite in my pancreas. For approximately nine months I had been suffering from chronic fatigue, hot sweats, broken sleep, bloating and skin rashes. Generally, I have a healthy diet, drink alcohol only in moderation, do not smoke and exercise regularly, and yet I could not beat the constant bouts of fatigue that were leaving me uninterested in life, emotional and very concerned about my health. The fatigue would be worse after exercise and my gradual weight gain was getting me down, not to mention the lack of focus on my work.

Susan explained that the parasite Giardia was often overlooked by doctors and yet could be present in many individuals. We discussed how I most likely contracted it from poor drinking water or close contact with a sick relative, and how such a small thing could have such a big effect on the human body. Susan gave me three bottles of 'magic potion', one to assist with my kidney function, one to repair my pancreas and a large bottle of wormwood, to kill the parasite. She also advised me to stay off gluten for a while as my stomach was struggling to digest it.

One week later I felt like a new person; friends commented on how well I looked. The rash on the back of my neck and forearms had significantly diminished, the hot sweats had gone and, most importantly, my energy levels had finally returned to normal. For the first time in a long time I felt normal again!

Susan was confident the parasite was no longer in my system and no further treatment was needed.

Three weeks on and I still feel great, my skin is continuing to improve, I have increased my levels of exercise and am finally getting control of my weight. As advised, I have continued to avoid gluten in my diet and I no longer have instant bloating after eating a meal. I continue to be amazed at how something (a parasite) so small, and that I had never even heard of before, could have caused me so many problems.

Summary

We have seen what a wide range of health imbalances a Giardia infestation can create, most of which would not normally be considered related to this parasite. From skin problems and sleep disturbance to teeth grinding and weight loss – the health checklist gives a clear indication of this unwelcome visitor's presence in the body.

It is really important not to ignore these signs – the consequences of an undiagnosed Giardia infestation are discussed in the next chapter.

Chapter 4

Gut reactions

The havoc Giardia can wreak on the human digestive system is significant and progressive. Once it has arrived in an unsuspecting host, it begins its damaging regime by flattening the tall, finger-like villi that protrude into the lumen of the small intestine, and which are essential for good nutritional health.

The villi increase the surface area for absorption, effectively extending the gut surface to the size of two or three football pitches. When Giardia damage the villi, absorption suffers, and about 50% of people I treat for giardiasis have already developed a gluten sensitivity as a result.

If those affected in this way continue to eat gluten, they may suffer bloating, diarrhoea, wind and nausea, and this can continue even after the Giardia have been destroyed. I always recommend avoiding gluten for the duration of treatment in these cases, otherwise there will be no improvement. Indeed, some people are better off *never* going back to gluten.

Sufferers of coeliac disease (an autoimmune reaction to gluten) should always avoid eating gluten, but I have treated patients who do not have coeliac disease and yet are only able to cope with their symptoms when following a coeliac diet. This is due to the presence of, and damage caused by, Giardia. Take the example of my patient 'James', who wrote the following about his own experience.

James's story

My gut problems started with a bout of serious diarrhoea that descended on me after I'd foolishly consumed a roadside smoothie on holiday in Istanbul. After that I was always getting tummy upsets, and produced a lot of gas. Tests for wheat and gluten allergies were inconclusive and my problem was put down to IBS, but my GP said he'd had another patient who had benefited from a gluten-free diet despite having test results like mine.

Going on a coeliac (gluten-free) diet, with the help of a nutritionist, made my symptoms more manageable, but I wasn't 100% problem free. A gastroenterologist said my test results for coeliac disease were 'very' negative, so gluten was obviously not the only culprit. It was only when I found Susan, and was tested for Giardia – three years after my gut problems had started – that I finally got the help I needed.

Susan talks about peeling back the layers of problems before getting to the core issue, and, in my case, it took three separate courses of herbs before I felt that my gut was really back to normal again.

I am now on a normal diet, without any problems, but I wonder how many other people diagnosed as IBS/coeliac in the UK have picked up a parasite but remain undiagnosed due to testing difficulties. I have since discovered that, although the Giardia lamblia parasite is widely distributed worldwide and easily transmitted (according to the World Health Organization), its identification in the UK is difficult using existing techniques.

Coeliac disease (CD)

According to Coeliac UK, an organisation set up to help those suffering from this disease, approximately one in 100 people have this condition.[1] As previously mentioned this is classed as an autoimmune disorder – where the immune system attacks the body and in this case causes an immunological response to gluten which can have devastating effects on the gut and beyond.

Symptoms include chronic diarrhoea, failure to thrive (in children) and fatigue, but sufferers can have CD and yet have none of these 'typical' symptoms. Some people have only a rash and, because they have no apparent digestive symptoms, their true condition can easily escape diagnosis. The condition is caused by a reaction to gliadin – a gluten-protein found in wheat – and to similar proteins found in barley and rye. Exposure to gliadin will cause an inflammatory reaction, which leads to destruction of the surface of the small intestine, known as villus atrophy. This can seriously affect nutritional health because the intestinal villi are responsible for absorption of nutrients. Without them we cannot get the benefit of what we eat.

If CD is suspected, a 'tissue transglutaminase Immunoglobulin antibody blood test', or 'tTG IgA', is done to help doctors diagnose the disease. By measuring the levels of antibody protein (IgA) in the blood sample, it can be determined whether the immune system is making antibodies to gliadin, which attack an enzyme in the intestines called tissue transglutaminase (iTG).

The results are not always conclusive, so a negative test does not always mean the patient does not have CD, but 98% of those suspected of having it, and who are on a diet containing gluten, will get a positive result to this test.

The only standardised known effective treatment for coeliac disease is a lifelong gluten-free diet.[2] But what if Giardia, not coeliac disease, was the cause of the gluten intolerance? It is entirely possible, because the Giardia parasite also damages the villi, as already discussed. However, the difference is that, following the elimination of the Giardia parasite, the gut lining can return to normal as referenced in the example below.

A study of a young child whose blood test for CD (IgA Anti-tTG) was positive, and who was suffering from severe diarrhoea and intestinal mucosa (gut lining) atrophy during a giardiasis infection, found his intestinal mucosa returned to normal after treatment for the giardiasis. Even though he no longer avoided gluten he remained symptom-free. It is very unusual for intestinal damage to right itself in patients with CD unless they are on a strict gluten-free diet.[3]

Whether diagnosed with CD, or simply feeling better on a gluten-free diet, there is a lot to take on board when trying to eliminate gluten from the diet because it is in such a wide variety of foods, and for those treading this path, any food that has been processed needs its label to be carefully scrutinised.

With approximately 50% of my Giardia patients developing a gluten sensitivity, I have provided some guidelines to help those in this situation and these can be found in Appendix III.

Penny's story

'Penny' was a patient struggling to manage her coeliac disease. Her attempts to control her exposure to gluten did not seem to be working because, despite her strict gluten-free diet, Penny's blood analysis showed her antibody markers were still rising. I diagnosed Penny with giardiasis, and treated her with Artemesia annua (wormwood). A few weeks later Penny contacted me to say:

As I mentioned, my tTg IgA antibody (95% specific to coeliac disease) has been on the increase instead of decrease despite my strict gluten-free diet.It rose steadily each time I had the tests (80, 85, 170) until in March when it went off the scale, literally, at 300+ (they stop measuring at 300). This antibody indicates damage to the intestine (rather than the presence of gluten). I had a set of tests done in May, three weeks after I took the wormwood and it had come down to 80, which was great but still a high positive; however, yesterday the result came back as 21!

That's considered 'weak positive' and is quite an amazing drop in such a short time. I can't tell you how delighted I am; there is no question for me that your treatment achieved this. I've done absolutely nothing different other than take that. So either the Giardia was keeping my intestines from responding to the gluten-free diet or, fingers crossed, it was nothing to do with gluten at all!

Good news number two is that my essential vitamin D, B12 and ferritin and mineral levels are now back to within normal ranges. My ferritin level was persistently critically low at around 7 -10 [nanograms per millilitre of blood ng/ml] for the last 18 months; it's now 33. Vitamin D is now up from 10 to 62 ng/ml (the higher end of normal) and B12 also from very low to 243 ng/ml. I am taking supplements for all of these and that has undoubtedly helped; however, I was not able to absorb them before and now, clearly, I am.

Lastly I have gained around 4 kilos in weight since I took the wormwood and am now back to my original weight, which again is just amazing!

Lactose intolerance

It is now clear that Giardia's negative impact on the gut, and its lining of villi, can impinge on the absorption of nutrients. It can also affect the production of essential digestive enzymes, such as lactase which is used to digest lactose, the natural sugar in milk. Even if a person is only temporarily affected, it can be distressing because, without lactase, undigested lactose ferments and causes cramping, bloating, diarrhoea and nausea.

People with full-blown lactose intolerance do not produce enough lactase, so have a constant problem with the sugars in dairy products, causing diarrhoea, flatulence, bloating, cramping and abdominal pain. If, however, these symptoms are temporary and caused by Giardia, they should clear up when the parasite has been destroyed.[4]

In an Italian study, children who had suffered from giardiasis were found to be prone to lactose malabsorption yet able to eat yoghurt.[5] Yoghurt has the ability to restore lactase activity in the intestine of children with *Giardia lamblia* infection[6] but only 'live' yoghurt, containing live bacteria, including microbial galactosidase (lactase) offers this benefit. Heated or pasteurised yoghurts do not contain the beneficial bacteria needed to prevent lactose malabsorption or symptoms of intolerance.[7]

Leaky gut syndrome and food allergies

When a parasite attaches itself to the intestinal wall it can increase the permeability of the gut, leading to a downward spiral of ill-health. The health problems it causes, mainly allergy and autoimmunity, arise from excessive absorption of antigens over-stimulating the immune response. The liver also becomes stressed as toxins, derived from the chemical activity of intestinal bacteria, are absorbed.

As well as inflammatory bowel symptoms, this process of inflammation can lead to arthritis, fatigue, migraines, food allergies and skin-related problems, such as eczema, hives and psoriasis.[8]

Vitamin B12 deficiency

Giardia can also cause malabsorption of vitamin B12, which is vital for the formation of red blood cells, as well as for the proper functioning of nerve tissue.[9]

If B12 deficiency continues and goes untreated over a period of time it can lead to damage to the brain, central and peripheral nervous systems, with any of the following as early symptoms:

- Tingling hands and feet
- Muscle weakness
- Difficulties with walking and coordination
- A diminished sense of touch.

Memory loss, confusion and depression may accompany any of the above symptoms, and tiredness, palpitations, a red, sore mouth and enlarged tongue, weight loss and diarrhoea are further signs.

In my early years of diagnosing giardiasis, I had a patient who was experiencing difficulty with her coordination. She could not swim due to her poor health and her walking was becoming a problem.

As part of her examination I tested her for Giardia, which proved positive. She was going on holiday that week and I gave her wormwood to take with her, and off she went. The following week, on her second visit, she said that she had swum for the first time in many years and felt so much better. This made me realise that Giardia could affect the nervous system and not just the digestive area.

I understand now that this lady must have had a B12 deficiency due to Giardia infestation, and it was the wormwood I prescribed that restored her gut lining to normality. Once she was able to absorb B12 again, all her symptoms disappeared very quickly.

However, it is important to be aware that the wormwood protocol does not work if any underlying digestive issues are not dealt with, as the following story explains.

Mary's story

Mary picked up Giardia whilst travelling in India in 2015. It caused her to feel sick, tired and dizzy. Her eyesight became jumpy and she lost weight and also saw her hair start to fall out. She was treated, and was symptom free after six months but, after another trip to India the following year, her illness returned with a vengeance. Her hair was falling out in big clumps, and she had terrible digestive issues.

This time she went to her GP, who admitted she knew nothing about Giardia and had to look it up before sending the recommended three stool samples off for analysis. The results came back a month later and were positive for Giardia. Mary started a course of the antibiotic metronidazole, which made no difference at all. After another test, two weeks later, and with a further positive reading for Giardia, she was then offered tinidazole, but declined as she felt so unwell on antibiotics. She tried various herbal remedies that she had researched herself before finding me and starting my treatment with wormwood. I also prescribed herbs for her gallbladder.

After a week on the treatment, she was convinced it wasn't working as she still felt unwell. However, she was drinking eight very large cups of tea (with soya milk) every day, and the tannins in tea are known to affect the gut lining, restricting the digestive process. Soya milk can also be indigestible. I was sure the Giardia had gone and that her digestive issues were the result of the excessive tea drinking and also her consumption of wheat, to which she was also sensitive. I advised her to cut these out. It was not easy for her to do this, but she then reported to me.

'I'm feeling so much better. My stomach has calmed down, my energy level has improved and I have little gas. I generally feel better than I have in four months. I have cut out wheat, tea, soya milk, soya food, processed food and dairy. I can only think I must be gluten sensitive.'

Mary had her test results back and told me:

'I am clear of Giardia and feeling better every day.'

Summary

Gluten sensitivity is greatly enhanced in many of my patients with a Giardia infestation, followed to a lesser degree by a lactose intolerance. Giardiasis can also mimic the effect on the microvilli of the gut lining that is seen in coeliac disease. In my view, this is reason enough for a Giardia infestation to be considered prior to a diagnosis of coeliac disease being given.

Stress also plays an important part in determining whether we are vulnerable to the havoc Giardia can cause within the body and the next chapter explains this in more detail.

Chapter 5

Giardia and stress

Having an undiagnosed Giardia infestation is very stressful for many people and as we have discussed, stress, left unchecked, can damage and weaken a healthy immune system. At the same time, a weakened immune system always leaves us open to illness and this would include parasitic infestation, so it is certainly possible for Giardia to take up residence in a person whose immune system is already under attack from chronic stress.

The full impact of having giardiasis and the stressful effect it can have on lives is best explained by Jane's story:

Jane's story

After being diagnosed for several years with irritable bowel syndrome (IBS), I turned to herbalist Susan Koten for help when the so-called IBS got out of control and began to rule my life and mind.

Always looking for a bathroom and having a constant feeling that I needed to rush to the toilet with violent diarrhoea became normal for me. Most people would think this would be stressful, but I assure you all that is an understatement.

- *Work: Simple things such as travelling to work had become a nightmare. Thirty minutes on a train with no toilet or, worse, a toilet available but the train so full of people in rush hour that you physically cannot walk to get into it. My palms*

*dripping with sweat while I wait to get off the train and
get to a toilet at my interchange station. Never being able
to complete my journey in full is my everyday nightmare.
Countless hours stuck at a station just because the toilet
was there and I could not put myself on a train without one,
to get home.*

- *Family occasions: My mother's birthday, having to leave a
  family afternoon tea and shopping day in London because
  my stomach was so bad I had to be near a toilet and
  could not browse shops – simple everyday things we take
  for granted were being ruled by what I now know was a
  parasite called Giardia.*

- *Holidays: Calling the airline ahead to pre-allocate me a seat
  near a toilet as the thought of a nine-hour flight petrified
  me. Going through passport control lines of 30 minutes I
  have had to walk out of to get to a toilet.*

*For a fact, I had a very delicate stomach, certainly had diarrhoea
and nausea daily, but I now know Giardia also causes stress
and anxiety even in the strongest of people. It's a vicious cycle
because you do have 'near accidents' if you can't get to a toilet
in time. You know you'll have stomach cramps daily that indicate
a need to go, but you can't control when or where this will
happen, so your mind starts to panic ahead daily.*

*My symptoms got so bad that one week I couldn't actually get
out of bed. I was so upset that I couldn't go out and do normal
things, scared to eat not knowing what my 'trigger' would be.
The effect this had on my professional status at work has been
overwhelming.*

*No one really understands unless they too have experienced
this. Some say it's 'in your mind', but the proof is shown daily
that it's not, when I'm in the toilet. Some say, 'Oh, just take
some Imodium.' Well, I did take whole packets some days, and
then I was doubled up with pain. Even if the diarrhoea stopped,
the cramps and nausea and sweats continued.*

*It's a total understatement to say that Giardia just affects you in
the gut, and even though my symptoms are almost gone I am
still very anxious about not being near a toilet.*

So what is stress?

Most people have their own view as to what stress is. Some think of it as the feelings they experience when stuck in a traffic jam on their way to pick up the children, or when going to an important meeting they now fear they will miss. It is normally associated with the sense of being out of control in some way.

Hans Selye, a Hungarian-Canadian endocrinologist, was the first person to identify stress as a medical term, and in 1936 he published his theory of the General Adaptation Syndrome (GAS), which explains three stages the body goes through when dealing with stress.[1] These are:

- alarm reaction
- resistance or adaptation
- exhaustion.

They can be summarised as follows:

Alarm reaction: This is when the 'fight or flight' mechanism in our body is triggered.

Resistance or adaption: This is when the body makes efforts to respond to the stress and begins secreting glucocorticoids (steroid hormones) to try and cope with the new situation. Cortisol is one such hormone and its job is to replenish the energy supplies, and manage the cardiovascular function, during this emergency.

Exhaustion: This is when the body can no longer fight against the stressors because of depletion of energy resources.

Since the 1930s when Hans Selye was coming up with his theories, stress has become a significant factor in modern life, and many people live with medium to high levels of stress on a daily basis. Many more take medication to control its negative effects.

We now know much more about the physical and emotional damage stress can cause if allowed to develop unchecked. It not only affects our relationships and our ability to function effectively at work, but it also has major consequences for our ability to cope with and get over illness, because chronic stress can and does negatively effect our immune system.

How the immune system reacts to stress

Our immune system is our body's first line of defence against bacteria, viruses, parasites, fungi and much more – it behaves in a similar way to a well-equipped, highly organised and effective army defending the human organism against all comers. It operates throughout the body and involves many types of cells, organs, proteins and tissues. Without a strong, healthy immune system our bodies become weak and soon fall prey to illness, chronic fatigue and, eventually, a shorter than expected life. The immune system is 'responsive', meaning it is activated when it detects a threat or any foreign invaders in the body and immediately gets to work creating and releasing the necessary antibodies, hormones and other biochemicals designed to defend it. However, there are other ways the immune system is activated also, and these can be more subtle triggers, as with stress.

Stress is not a pathogen, or a virus, or any other external threat, but as we already know, it is a very real issue when it comes to health and, if not addressed, will very soon suppress the immune system and leave the body unprotected and vulnerable to all these external threats.

Stress has a positive place in the human story and it played a primal role in keeping us alive in our primitive past. The 'fight or flight' response we have to danger helped ensure the human species survived. When early humans were faced with a dangerous (stressful) situation, the brain and many systems in the body were immediately activated and heart rate, breathing, and blood pressure all increased. The endocrine system would release hormones such as cortisol and adrenaline pushing blood to the large muscle groups to provide the massive surge of energy needed to make a hasty getaway from the danger. At the same time, the immune system would become activated and immediately start releasing chemicals to ward off invaders, and all of these reactions were designed to deal with acute, rather than chronic, danger. Once the threat was gone, the body's chemistry would return to normal together with all the other systems – gut function, heart rate, breathing, etc.

Today, we have not evolved sufficiently to differentiate between true danger and perceived danger, and this system still operates very successfully in our bodies when we find ourselves in dangerous (stressful) situations such as taking an important exam, meeting a critical deadline at work, or receiving an enormous tax bill we weren't expecting.

Unfortunately, the stress problems we face today are chronic in many cases, and keeping the body in a permanent state of 'fight or flight' can injure the immune system and have serious consequences for our ongoing health.[2] It means effectively the 'army' is in a permanent state of readiness for action. Over time, the adrenal glands become exhausted and, while cortisol levels continue to rise, the most profound effect of adrenal exhaustion is the glands' waning ability to produce dehydroepiandrosterone (DHEA), the hormone designed to help restore normality after a period of stress. As DHEA falls, cortisol and adrenalin levels begin to fluctuate as well, as the adrenal glands attempt to meet increasingly impossible demands for more support.

Recognising symptoms of stress

We all know the feeling of sickness, butterflies, or urgently needing to empty our bowels when something upsets or shocks us, or when we face an ordeal such as a job interview or exam. These reactions are usually shortlived experiences of acute stress, and a healthy immune system can cope well with these situations until they are over and normal regulation of the body returns. However, illness, injury and dysfunctional relationships can stress the body in various ways, as can fear, grief and trauma (old or recent), yet it comes as a surprise to many people coping with such issues, that they are chronically stressed. The symptoms have become such a feature of their lives they do not see them as being abnormal. They may actually take comfort from the feeling that their heart is racing because it is what feels normal!

In my clinical practice, when treating giardiasis, I have often wondered why it is that, out of two people who are living together and sharing everything, only one of them may become infected with the Giardia parasite while the other remains free from infestation. They have seemingly eaten the same food, shared the same towels and drunk the same water, so what is it that singles out one person from the other?

I am convinced it has a lot to do with stress and a person's ability to successfully deal with it so it does not become a health issue. I have often observed that one partner is more stressed, or holds onto stress more rigidly, than the other; no prizes then for guessing it is the stressed one who generally is more prone to getting giardiasis.

The following is a list of symptoms associated with chronic stress, informed by Anxiety UK's information:[3]

- Periods of irritability or anger
- Apathy or depression
- Frequent crying
- Nail biting
- Loss of appetite
- Comfort eating
- Lack of concentration
- Loss of sex drive

- Increased smoking, drinking or taking recreational drugs
- Excessive tiredness
- Insomnia
- Aches and pains in muscles
- Heart palpitations and chest pain
- Feeling sick
- Stomach pain
- Weight loss or gain.

With a Giardia infestation not only can there be symptoms of bowel dysfunction, but these symptoms can lead to additional symptoms of stress which can include some or all of the above, as shown in Jane's story. Giardia loves Jane and her stressful condition. While she is constantly under stress, cortisol is being released, which, unchecked, lowers her immune system and flushes her body with glucose. This is the ideal environment for Giardia, as it feeds on glucose and is able to survive and flourish when the immune system is compromised. Stress has become a chronic complaint in our modern world for all sorts of reasons and unfortunately Giardia is adding to the problem by taking advantage of the perfect breeding and feeding ground for its existence.

Giardia feeds stress

Having a Giardia infestation can be an extremely stressful process in itself, as patients battle to get the right diagnosis. After conventional treatment for giardiasis, many patients come to me still complaining of digestive issues that their GP has grouped and labelled as being 'stress-related'.

I treated one man from New Zealand who had come to work in the UK for a few months. He was displaying many of the gut and bowel symptoms typical of giardiasis. I identified he was infested with Giardia and treated him until he was free of the parasite. However, upon his return to New Zealand, his symptoms came back. His doctor did not believe that he had Giardia and presumed his gut problems were psychological; he asked the man, 'Do you have girlfriend problems?'

My patient had to persuade the doctor to get him tested, and, as the test was not available in New Zealand, his samples had to be sent to Australia for diagnosis. The result confirmed the Giardia had returned, and, fortunately for my patient, a business trip brought him back to the UK so I was able to treat him with more herbs that this time cleared the problem up long term.

Most physical stress responses are accompanied by emotional responses and, as previously discussed, prolonged stress causes tension, irritability, short temperedness and increased anxiety. A Giardia infestation, and the disruption it causes, can continue for many years – a Norwegian study found a high prevalence of IBS and chronic fatigue diagnoses, three years after patients had suffered acute giardiasis.[4] The physical unpleasantness of wind, bloating, pain and generalised discomfort, together with, in some cases, severe and uncontrollable diarrhoea, will trigger an emotional response such as fear, anxiety, worry, panic and feelings of helplessness. Patients may also experience an inability to concentrate, think clearly, or remember information accurately, which are common cognitive reactions to stress. Stress may affect facial expression and body posture too because pain and misery cause people to stoop or frown as they begin to 'close down' under the weight of their worsening circumstances.

Those who perceive their illness as a challenge rather than a threat often experience fewer effects. How a patient perceives the positive or negative impact of their Giardia symptoms may also determine the impact stress has on them. If, however, stress does become an issue, it is very important for sufferers to take control of the Giardia quickly in order to help lower their stress levels and deal with the infestation swiftly.

Alison's story

Alison found it difficult to pinpoint exactly when, but she had started to notice subtle changes in her health. During our first consultation I found her immune system was not working optimally. She says:

I was experiencing tiredness and lack of concentration, and I had also begun to struggle with maintaining my weight. A year on and I was still battling with these symptoms, but I had also had difficulty sleeping and was experiencing changes in my menstrual cycle. I was worried enough to visit my GP, who within 30 seconds had diagnosed that I was most likely suffering from stress. I could not ignore what the doctor had said; my symptoms fitted the diagnosis, but other than the fast-paced demands of modern-day living, I did not feel that I was in any stressful situations that would be affecting my health. A year passed, and it was a huge effort to get up in the mornings. I had to alter my daily routine so that I could rest before I drove home after work, for fear of falling asleep whilst at the wheel. I was forever cancelling evening arrangements in favour of an early night. I lacked energy, and no amount of sleep was enough to rejuvenate me to complete daily tasks. This was when I began to feel like it was my fault, and that I was weak, as I looked at friends and family who were in far more stressful situations than me and they were still able to live their lives fully. Ten months later and I had got myself into a cycle of sleep, caffeine, sugar and – most nights – alcohol to get me through the working week. I had quit my Saturday job as I did not have the energy and I had been transformed from a fitness fanatic who had run a marathon the previous year into a couch potato. Despite receiving two promotions at work I was so uptight and anxious about people thinking I was stressed and not coping, that I put all of my limited energy into work. As a result, my confidence was low, my energy was low, my healthy lifestyle had been abandoned and I had completely lost my work-life balance. I reached the point where I could not continue. I became tearful and exhausted.

My GP diagnosed me with anxiety and depression and signed me off work. I was so desperate to feel better that I took the antidepressants he had prescribed, without hesitation. For six weeks I slept, and at no point did I feel that the medication was making me better; it was just suppressing my emotions. I was advised to speak with counsellors to learn to deal with my stress, anxiety and depression. I had initial consultations with two counsellors who both told me that I seemed very rational and clear in my thoughts, and that I did not need to see them again unless I felt the need to.

I felt completely lost at this point. I had left a job that I loved, I had become devoid of emotion, and I had professionals telling me that I was not experiencing the psychological issues that most patients with depression and anxiety show. I was determined to re-build my life, and after four months I stopped taking the medication. I took on board advice from anyone and everyone about what precautions I should take to prevent becoming stressed or depressed again. I must add at this point the most horrific and stressful experience by far was leaving my job and the lack of self-worth I had to battle with, believing that I was unable to cope. Nonetheless, I wanted to get my life back on track and re-training whilst planning to start a family was a decision that made me and my husband happy. Despite making every adjustment possible to my lifestyle it was not long before I was in exactly the same situation as I had been before, except this time I was scared. I did not know where to turn, and I was starting to worry that something was seriously wrong with me. I knew that if I went back to my GP I would tick every box for a relapse, but the crippling fatigue and irregular periods meant that I would not be able to fall pregnant anytime soon. The GP was slightly puzzled when I refused to accept stress or depression as a diagnosis. Instead he opted for blood tests, and when the results did not show any abnormalities, he just recommended that I monitor my situation. If I had not been directed to Susan's practice at this time, I fear for what might have happened to me. I was hanging on to life by my fingertips. I knew something was not right and I could not bear to carry on the way I was feeling with no guarantee that I would get better. I felt that I had completely lost control of my life and myself, which was a terrifying situation to be in. I visited Susan's clinic and, while I have always been open-minded about alternative *therapies, I was just in such a rut I did not think that anybody would be able to help me. Before diagnosis had even begun Susan was able to give me help that I had not received from anywhere else. She was not just interested in my symptoms, but in me as a whole person. After Susan's diagnosis of Giardia, I was given herbal supplements to destroy the parasite. The moment I left Susan's clinic the constant spotting I had been experiencing stopped, and by the next day I was able to think more clearly and stay awake for a whole day without needing to rest. For the first time in years I felt more like myself, my confidence and personality returned so quickly. I was making social arrangements, as well as keeping on top of household tasks, exercising and eating well. With the dietary guidance and lifestyle adjustments that Susan has recommended, I am sure I will be able to continue taking positive steps forward.*

I am overwhelmed by the progress I have made under the care and direction of Susan. If I had not been lucky enough to find Susan's practice when I did I would be in the process of getting a diagnosis for chronic fatigue syndrome. This would have taken such a long time, and I would have endured so much more unnecessary suffering. I only hope by sharing my experience that other people may benefit.

A few months later I had a follow-up call from Alison saying:

I just wanted to let you know that since receiving your treatment I have gone from strength to strength. My health and wellbeing improved so rapidly that I have been fortunate enough to fall pregnant without any difficulties. Our baby is due in six months and we are absolutely delighted. Thank you so much for your care and support.

Summary

An undiagnosed Giardia infestation can create stress and anxiety in the lives of many individuals as they try to cope with an array of seemingly unconnected symptoms. As shown in earlier chapters, the constant stress and worry of trying to get on with life in these circumstances can cause additional complications as the immune system can become compromised. This situation not only allows the undetected Giardia to flourish, but it also opens up opportunities for other organisms to invade and further weaken an already vulnerable system.

In the next chapter we look at how Giardia can invade the gut microbiome and the impact this can have on our wellbeing.

Chapter 6

Giardia and our natural defence barrier

In this chapter we will look at what nature provides in the way of protection for us from the unfriendly pathogens we will likely ingest or be exposed to in life, including Giardia.

The microbiome

The microbiome is the term used to describe the genetic material of all the microbes – bacteria, fungi, protozoa and viruses – that live on and inside the human body. Whilst some bacteria and other micro-organisms are associated with disease ('pathogens'), others are actually extremely important, not only for our immune system, but also for many other aspects of our overall health.

The digestive tract is home to trillions of these helpful bacteria and other microbes (the 'microbiota'), which colonise the gut and create an ecosystem called the 'gut microbiome'. An imbalance of the microbiota in the gut can cause gastrointestinal disturbances which have been linked to a number of chronic complaints, including irritable bowel syndrome (IBS) and inflammatory bowel disease (IBD). In order for Giardia to reach the epithelial cells that line the gut, where the parasite can gorge on the nutrients that *we* should be absorbing, it has to get through the gut microbiota and also the 'mucus barrier'.[1]

The mucus barrier

The entire gastrointestinal tract is coated inside with a thick layer of mucus which protects the underlying epithelial cells from pathogens and foreign particles that we may have inadvertently consumed. A variety of microbes live here and form a 'biofilm', like a protective envelope, to keep the environment healthy. Giardia have the ability to disrupt this biofilm.

The mucus also creates lubrication for the downward movement of foods, and its thickness increases through the gut, towards the colon. When Giardia get through this mucus barrier, they can access the epithelial cells and attach to them with their ventral discs, so feeding can begin unabated.

Factors for a healthy gut flora composition

Beneficial bacteria in the gut provide a natural barrier and protect against pathogenic bacteria, parasites, fungi, viruses and toxins, all of which are in the food we eat, the air we breathe and the water we drink. Apart from providing this physical barrier, the beneficial bacteria produce antibiotic-like substances that are antifungal and antiviral, thereby providing protection against various diseases.

The beneficial bacteria also help in the digestion and absorption of our food, and produce a number of enzymes that break down proteins, carbohydrates, fibre and fats. They produce various substances that transport vitamins, minerals and other nutrients from our food, through the gut wall, which are then absorbed into our blood stream. So, without a good, healthy gut flora, the body will be deficient in nutrients, simply because they cannot be absorbed properly.

The main members of our indigenous friendly bacteria are: bifidobacteria (*Bifidobacterium bifidum*), lactobacteria (*Lactobacillus acidophilus, Lactobacillus plantarum, Lactobacillus rhamnosus*), peptostreptococci and enterococci. 'Probiotic' is the term used to describe these beneficial micro-organisms, and they additionally help to crowd out harmful bacteria.

Disruptions to the balance of probiotics in the gut, such as an infestation of Giardia, can compromise the beneficial role they play in the body. People with an imbalance of probiotics and pathogens in the gut may experience poor digestion, lowered natural immunity and a large variety of conditions such as:

Low energy levels

Poor immunity

Gas or bloating

Food intolerances or allergies

Indigestion

Heartburn

Constipation or diarrhoea

Thrush and/or candida overgrowth

IBS (irritable bowel syndrome)

IBD (inflammatory bowel disease)

Acne and/or eczema.

An individual's gut flora will affect how Giardia establishes itself and may well influence the severity of the attack and the susceptibility to re-infection.[1]

Formation of a healthy microbiome

Let us take a look at how the microbiome is formed. One of the major factors in determining the health and strength of the gut flora is the way in which an individual comes into this world. A baby born naturally, via the vagina, is coated in the mother's microbiota, as it leaves the sterile environment of the womb and travels through the tight confines of the birth canal. Every orifice of the newborn, and its skin, gets smothered in this gloopy matter and this process sets them up with protection for entry into their new environment.[2]

Studies have shown that infants born through caesarean section do not get this early protection and their first exposure is to bacteria from the hospital environment and healthcare workers. However, although caesarean babies have shown less microbiota formation after one month, this seems to normalise after six months.[3]

Breast-fed infants also have less *Clostridium difficile* and *Escherichia coli* (harmful bacteria) in their intestinal tract than formula-fed infants, and it is becoming clearer, as more research is done, that the role of the mother in these early stages of life, and in particular for providing the building blocks for a healthy immune system, is even more important than had previously been thought.[4]

Giardia in pregnancy

Giardiasis affects people of all ages, and at all stages of life. It is, therefore, important to discuss its impact during pregnancy, and also on a new-born baby. Normally, giardiasis does not adversely affect a pregnancy, although the health of the mother is crucial during this time if the outcome is to be successful. For pregnant women who do become infected with this parasite, and experience nutritional malabsorption and weight loss, the infection could have a negative effect on their overall wellbeing and therefore the pregnancy.

A pregnant woman who becomes infected will find many of the prescribed drugs used to treat giardiasis are not safe to take during pregnancy, so it is likely the doctor will delay treatment until after the baby is born. However, when my daughter was pregnant with one of her babies she had digestive issues, and tested positive to Giardia. We used my Giardia herbal spray containing wormwood, which worked perfectly well and with no side effects. My herbal sprays are non-invasive, and work energetically (see Chapter 12). It is worth mentioning here that wormwood should not be taken internally during pregnancy and a pregnant woman wanting to ingest the herb to treat giardiasis should wait until after the birth and until she has finished breastfeeding.

Mums-to-be who have a diagnosed Giardia infestation should always keep their doctor updated on its effects, especially if they are dehydrated, have blood in their faeces, or have experienced bouts of diarrhoea or any other debilitating complication for longer than two weeks.

Giardia and children

Mums who are infected with the Giardia parasite may worry their baby will catch it from them when they breastfeed. Asymptomatic infections from Giardia or other parasites can occur during pregnancy, but it is thought these are not transmitted via breast milk to suckling babies. Recent research on the subject of breastfeeding and Giardia points out there are anti-Giardia factors in breast milk that prevent infection becoming established.[5]

The only other possible route of infection through breastfeeding would be via the nipple if the mother inadvertently carries Giardia on her fingers as she guides the nipple into the baby's mouth. However, if infection was transmitted to the baby via this route, the content of the breast milk and the protection it provides would enhance the infant's immunity against infection.

Although infection is rare during the first six months of life in breastfed infants, older infants and young children have an increased susceptibility to giardiasis, especially through exposure at day-care centres and schools, so the importance of hygiene when dealing with young children (especially if regularly changing nappies) cannot be overstated.

Children can pick up infection just as easily as adults and

the symptoms will be there to see if the parents are aware. An infected child can appear not to be thriving and to be sickly and distressed, complaining of headaches, stomach pains, feeling nauseous and maybe teeth grinding. Constipation and/ or diarrhoea are very likely too. Of course, these symptoms can be caused by a number of other conditions as well, but if they persist and become debilitating, a Giardia infestation will definitely need to be ruled out.

One mother described her six-year-old son, who had become infected, as being out of control and hyperactive. After taking the herbs I prescribed, the child's behaviour settled back to normal (wormwood should always be prescribed by a herbal practitioner and not self-medicated). My Giardia remedy can be sprayed externally and is not ingested so there is no potential battle for children to take medicines and, as it bypasses the digestive system, no nasty taste or side effects. Sprays are quick, easy and simple to use and children do not seem to mind them at all, which is a blessing. My daughter uses herbal sprays I mix for all her children's ailments.

Even a five year old can be labelled with IBS – this is Becky's story (not her real name) as told by her mother.

Becky's story

I remember the exact point my daughter Becky started having stomach problems. She was three and a half and we were at a holiday camp in the UK. She started complaining of stomach pains after her meals and would be doubled up in pain. She then developed a really high temperature. I took her to the doctor and he said she had some type of virus. The virus only lasted for a few days but from that point onwards all Becky's problems began. She continued to be doubled up in pain after every meal. She had a very bloated tummy and lots of painful wind. The doctor prescribed laxatives as he thought it was constipation. These did not help. We started experimenting with her diet. We cut out all dairy and this seemed to help at first. Then it started getting worse again, so we cut out all wheat. Again, this helped for a while but then it started getting worse again. By this time, we were referred to a consultant specialising in paediatric abdominal problems. She tested Becky for lactose intolerance and coeliac disease. The test results were negative. Becky was also complaining of a painful leg and feeling tired all the time. The consultant explained to us she did not know what the problem was and labelled it under the very general diagnosis of irritable bowel syndrome (IBS).

Becky started to get worse again and we noticed that the problems occurred after she had eaten fruit or anything containing sugar. We took Becky to a nutritionist. We were asked to compile a food diary of everything Becky ate and list any effects afterwards. After studying this list, the nutritionist advised us that we also needed to cut out all glucose from Becky's diet. This included most fruits and many vegetables as they all contained glucose. She was able to have fruits that only contained fructose, such as grapes, conference pears and cantaloupe melon. Becky was now on an extremely restricted diet, which was really tough for her. We had had to cut out dairy, wheat and glucose. It was very difficult to maintain and also very expensive and time-consuming to prepare separate meals for her. Every now and then we would try and introduce foods back into her diet, but she would just be doubled up in pain.

We struggled on like this until just before Becky's fifth birthday. My father then read an article in the Telegraph about a lady who seemed to have had the same problems as Becky was having for years. She had visited Susan Koten at the Willow Herbal Centre, who had diagnosed that she had contracted Giardia lamblia. The lady in the article said that Susan had cured her problem and transformed her life. I rang and made an appointment immediately. I took Becky for her appointment. Susan confirmed that Becky did indeed have Giardia and that I also had it. She advised that the rest of the family probably had been infected too, so we would all need to be treated. She explained that she would normally prescribe a tincture of a herb called wormwood. She, however, decided against this as I was still breastfeeding my son at the time. Instead, she made up the tincture into a spray. We were instructed to spray ourselves every day for a week. After a week we all visited Susan for another appointment. She told us we were all clear of Giardia. Tentatively at first, we started introducing foods back into Becky's diet. She had no problems and within a very short amount of time she was eating without any restrictions. We were absolutely amazed. We are so grateful to my lovely late father who found the article in the Telegraph as without that, we would probably still be in the same position today. But most importantly, we are hugely grateful to Susan for making such a difference to Becky's life.

I cannot understand why, after so many trips to doctors and specialists, that none of them mentioned Giardia and wonder how many more people have been misdiagnosed and are suffering as a result.

Poor diet

For us to be alive and healthy, we need to eat foods that are also alive and healthy. Unfortunately, modern life and our desire to charge through it at the speed of light, leaves little time for careful shopping, food preparation and cooking. Our dependence on commercially provided prepacked food hands the job of looking after our own health to large corporations who tempt us to buy their products with clever marketing, cheap ingredients and ease of use.

As a result, we have developed a love affair with sugar and many people are addicted to sweet foods. A leisurely stroll down the aisles of any supermarket reveals rows and rows of sugar-laden products in the form of cereals, soft drinks, wines, breads, biscuits, cakes, jams, chocolates and sweets. But a diet of cakes, biscuits, sweets and fruit juices, together with sugary prepackaged meals, soft fizzy drinks and wine puts a strain on the pancreas, and over a period of time may cause a person to develop type 2 diabetes, obesity, skin problems, fatigue, constipation, cataracts, oedema, candida and any number of related digestive issues. The list goes on and on and we must also include parasitic infestations, such as Giardia, because they also love a sweet environment and seem to do so well in it!

This addiction to sugar also creates other adverse effects. Dr Linus Pauling, the man who discovered vitamin C which helps to combat the common cold, also discovered that sugar severely slows down this process.[6]

Adding to this observation, another researcher, Dr John Ely, came up with the glucose-ascorbate-antagonism (GAA) theory which basically proposes glucose and vitamin C (both sharing a similar chemical make-up) compete to enter the body's cells, with glucose effectively restricting the amount of vitamin C a cell can receive. So, eating a high-sugar diet not only competes with our ability to absorb and use vitamin C, but also creates the ideal habitat for Giardia and other parasities, worms and fungi to thrive.

In my view, maintaining a strong and healthy gut microbiome is key to good health, and I have provided further reading material on how to do this in Appendix IV (page 151).

Summary

The microbiota which colonise the gut create an ecosystem called the gut microbiome. This ecosystem is a major component of our immune system. Giardia are adept at plundering our nutrients at cellular level, disrupting this gut microbiome and, thereby, affecting the health of the host – that's us.

The formation of the microbiome starts at birth and determines how healthy and strong our immune system will be throughout life. Children can be at risk of picking up Giardia and becoming prey to allergies and food intolerances, as discussed in the next chapter.

Chapter 7

Allergies

The impact a Giardia infestation can have on a person will vary according to the person's age and the state of their immune system at the time of infestation. If they are lucky, their symptoms will be mild and, with treatment, should be of short duration. However, even with a strong immune system, infestation, if left undiagnosed, can become chronic, during which time the parasite's ability to damage the gut lining and inferfere with the absorption of nutrients, plus the ramifications that will bring, will weaken the host's ability to produce antibodies to destroy it.

The immune system has within its armoury white blood cells called 'mast' cells which play an important part in detecting and dealing with pathogens attacking and invading the body. These cells are everywhere in our bodies and will respond immediately to any threat, inside or out, perceived or otherwise. Mast cells have the capacity to kill or call up the necessary substances to deal with any invader, and allergens such as pollen, dust mites and cat dander, are viewed by them as a threat. When mast cells are triggered, they will immediately start to release biochemicals such as histamine. These chemicals are called 'mediators' and are part of the inflammatory process that helps the immune system deal with 'enemies', producing the typical symptoms we associate with allergy. The role of mast cells in relation to giardiasis and the exacerbation of allergies during infection is still unclear, but scientific studies using mice show a connection between heightened allergic reactions and the presence of *Giardia lamblia*.[1]

During a Giardia infestation, the immune system has to constantly create different antibodies to fight the parasite, as it regularly alters its appearance, by switching its surface proteins to avoid detection. Meanwhile, allergic responses to foods and other substances become far more likely, as allergens penetrate through the damaged gut lining – responses which did not exist prior to the infestation.

Millions of people are affected by allergies in the UK. Unfortunately, the number is rising by 5% each year, and half of those affected are children according to Allergy UK.[2] Hay fever is the commonest allergy, but pet dander, foods, moulds and tree pollen also produce the same symptoms of sneezing, wheezing and nasal congestion.

I have noticed when I treat giardiasis, some allergy symptoms reduce, and asthma symptoms can also improve considerably. Many food allergies disappear too. It is no coincidence that studies have shown a clear relationship between giardiasis and allergy, possibly because the infection increases sensitivity towards food antigens, as concluded in a study of children infected with Giardia, of whom 70% had allergy symptoms.[3]

Let us take a closer look at allergies, and how Giardia can affect them.

Asthma

According to Allergy UK, there are 5.4 million people with asthma in the UK – that is, around one in 12 adults and one in 11 children being treated for asthma. The overall figure for Ireland is thought to be one in eight people. It is estimated that, by 2025, 400 million people worldwide will be suffering from this chronic complaint.[4]

The condition is characterised by difficulty breathing, and patients experience wheezing and coughing. Asthmatic people tend to breathe shallowly and rapidly through the mouth. Their posture is often stooped, with rounded shoulders, as if protecting the front part of their body from attack or exposure to the elements, but this posture also restricts their breathing, exacerbating the problem. On top of that, there is usually a tendency to hyperventilate, gulping at air as if they cannot get enough of it. This can dry out the airways, causing the sufferer to overdose the body on oxygen, irritating and constricting the breathing passages further.

In my practice I have seen how Giardia can exacerbate asthma. It is this immunological hypersensitivity to *Giardia lamblia* that has been shown to cause the irritation that precedes an asthma attack, according to the doctor and author Leo Galland MD.[5]

Killing off the Giardia can bring remission from asthma, which will be music to the ears of many people who have been told their condition will require a lifetime of medication with steroid inhalers. Unfortunately, steroids, taken over the long term, can contribute to vitamin and mineral deficiency, bone loss, and even diabetes.[6] Allergy medications also increase the risk of infection and reduce the immune system's ability to fight pathogenic invaders so, for many reasons, I believe those patients suffering from asthma could benefit from a test to establish if Giardia is present in their gut.

Tom's story

I initially came to Susan's centre with my fiancée as she was suffering from a bowel/stomach problem. My only reason for coming was to give her support. I had never believed in herbal medicine and to be honest I did not think Susan would be able to help her. My fiancée had suffered from constipation for many years and about two months prior to coming to Susan's office she had been suffering severe cramps and a bloated stomach. She had gone to her GP who advised her to take Senokot. She had taken many of these remedies, including laxatives and Buscopan, in the past which had only provided short-term relief. Eventually she insisted on being referred to a bowel specialist and the referral was made.

When Susan started muscle-testing my fiancée and noticed the weakness in her gallbladder, and said it was a parasite because her arm started moving to the smallest touch, I thought it was crazy. (I did not really believe Susan was doing anything!) It wasn't until Susan asked me to hold her hand, and did it again – that was when my arm started moving! To be honest, it freaked me out because I was trying everything to hold it in one place but I was not able to. I knew then that what Susan was doing was real. She said my fiancée was gluten-intolerant and gave her some herbs to take away. One week later there was a major improvement and after two weeks she was back to her normal self and had no problems. To date she has not had to take anything for her stomach and has not suffered any pain; she is very happy!

On her second visit we started chatting about my asthma so Susan decided to do the muscle test on me, which showed a weakness on my chest. She suggested I take the herbs to get rid of the parasite which could potentially give asthma-like symptoms. I had been diagnosed by my GP at the age of seven with asthma; I am now 31. The cause of my developing asthma was put down to the fact that we got a puppy when I was a child. I have taken Seretide and Salbutamol for many years, never knowing what they were actually doing to my health; the asthma never improved in any way. The first few days of taking the herbs I felt my chest clearing; I stopped using my pumps from that day. Unfortunately, due to the bad weather, I later got a chest infection which did make me a bit short of breath, so I have used my pumps occasionally but definitely not as much as I used to, which is a major improvement – thank you Susan for your help!

Allergic rhinitis

The term 'allergic rhinitis' covers the runny-nose symptoms produced by both indoor allergens, such as dust mites and pet dander, and outdoor allergens like grass pollen, mould spores and tree pollen.

I have noticed that patients with hay fever/allergic rhinitis respond well after being treated with herbs for giardiasis and have less of a reaction to pollens, grasses and other allergens.

Hay fever is an allergic reaction to pollens that floods the bloodstream with 'histamine'; this in turn inflames the nasal passages, causing the sinus lining to swell as it tries to get rid of the problem. This swelling can clog the delicate sinus membranes and damage the cilia – tiny delicate hairs that line the sinuses and move the watery mucus through the nasal passages, keeping them moist and clear of debris.

Pollens are generally released from March through to November, and the timing of the symptoms should give a clue to which pollens cause the problem. In spring (late March to mid-May) it may be tree pollens, in summer (mid-May to July) grasses (about nine out of 10 sufferers are allergic to grass pollen), and in autumn, fungi.

For those suffering all year round (known as 'perennial allergic rhinitis'), house dust mites are high on the list for consideration. Constant bouts of sneezing indoors, itchy eyes, nose and/or throat and possible cough, are all symptoms of this allergy. Feathers or animal dander may also be the culprit as they can produce similar symptoms. Cushions, pillows and duvets should be checked to make sure these are filled with hypoallergenic materials.

Allergies and the sinuses

As previously mentioned, allergies can play havoc with the sinuses, and create blockages of mucus in these delicate membranes, as they struggle to clear away debris. This then sets up problems in the ears, nose, head and eyes. During my travels to India I was shown a cleansing programme called 'Kriya', which I have passed on to my patients who have found it very effective in clearing their sinuses.

1. Take a cup of boiling water and let this cool to blood temperature. (Test the temperature by pouring some over the back of your hand; it should feel very comfortable.) To this tepid water add a good pinch of salt and stir it in. Pour a small amount of this solution into the right cupped hand.

2. Next, using the index finger of the left hand, close off the left nostril airway, and sniff the mixture up through the right nostril from the right cupped hand.

3. Snort out the sniffed contents with three hearty snorts then repeat the same process with the left hand and right nostril.

4. Slowly draw the palm of the right hand across the forehead and then the left-hand palm across the forehead – repeat each hand action three times.

5. Using the index and third finger, locate the bony projections of the cheekbones, follow the line of the cheekbones down to the back of the upper teeth and push them up towards the temple. Repeat three times.

6. Place the fingertips of each hand at the back of the jaw bone and push upwards, separating the ring and little finger in front of the ear and the index and middle finger behind the ear, forming a V-shape which stops when the earlobe is in the base of the V of the fingers. Move this up to the earlobe and back to the jaw base three times.

This process massages the sinus areas of the face and is very therapeutic and relaxing for the facial muscles as well as for clearing the sinuses.

If there is infection, this cleanse may be done every morning until the condition has cleared. Otherwise, one or two times each week as part of a cleansing routine is sufficient. Do not lie down for at least half an hour after completing this process just to make sure all the solution has drained out of the sinuses.

Note that salt can be very drying and may irritate the lining of the nose – if this becomes a problem discontinue using the cleanse.

Mould allergy

Mould spores can also trigger allergy symptoms. They come from sources such as rotting food, fungi and black mould on window frames or damp places in buildings. Some mould spores are seasonal whilst others are in the air all year round. Mould showed up as a problem when I was muscle testing one of my patients, but he could not think of any cause. Eventually, a few months later, he had been going to replace his mobile phone and had opened the back to remove its sim card, only to find the inside of the phone full of black mould! He knew that some time before he had dropped the phone in some water, but he thought he had dried it out. In fact, for months he had been breathing in spores from this mould, every time he made a phone call!

Food intolerances and allergies

When Giardia trophozoites attach themselves to the duodenum and jejenum, they interfere with the normal absorption of nutrients, as I have said, and this can play a part in causing food allergies and intolerances. A food intolerance occurs when the gut is unable to properly process or breakdown certain foods –

for example, lactose, the sugar that is found in milk and other dairy products. A food intolerance is much more common than a food allergy and takes hours rather than minutes for symptoms to develop. Symptoms of food intolerance include irritable bowel syndrome (IBS) and bloating, but also fatigue, eczema and rashes as well as migraine and even myalgic encephalomyelitis (ME), chronic fatigue syndrome (CFS), ulcerative colitis and rheumatoid arthritis.

Food allergies involve a much quicker response. When the body is exposed to a food it considers harmful, the immune system is galvanised into action and creates antibodies to fight it. When the particular food is eaten again, these antibodies, known as immunoglobulin E (IgE), are released along with histamine and other chemicals, in order to deal with the threat this substance represents.

Allergy symptoms range from minor to severe, with the worst outcome being anaphylactic shock – an extreme, often life-threatening allergic reaction to an antigen to which the body has become hypersensitive. Reactions usually happen as soon as the culprit food has been eaten and can include abdominal pain, itchy skin, hives, rashes, runny nose, wheezing, shortness of breath and a range of other symptoms as the body tries to get rid of the problem. Common food allergens include peanuts, fish, including shellfish, milk, eggs, soya products and wheat.

Wheat allergy

A wheat allergy can cause the immune system to react to any of the four groups of wheat protein – namely, albumin, globulin, gliadin and gluten – with typical symptoms ranging from irritation in the mouth and throat to headache, stomach cramps and again, anaphylactic shock.

Clearly the best way to deal with a wheat allergy is to avoid wheat products. The obvious culprits are pasta, many breads, biscuits, cakes and other baked goods, but many other foods contain wheat flour so those with this particular allergy should carefully check all their food labels.

Giardia and allergic skin problems

Urticaria

Urticaria (also known as hives or nettle rash) is a reaction to histamine that causes an itchy, raised rash anywhere on the skin and an outbreak can be caused by Giardia infestation.[7]

With acute urticaria, the wheals on the skin usually come in self-limiting bouts of less than 24 hours, over the course of several weeks. An attack will usually be caused by foods such as nuts, chocolate, fish, tomatoes, eggs, fresh berries, soya, wheat and milk, or by medicines, infections, insect bites or internal disease. However, chronic urticaria, can last for six weeks or more; thankfully, if Giardia is the cause and is successfully treated, then the urticaria will also abate.

Angioedema

Angioedema is a swelling caused by a build-up of fluid in deeper layers of the skin, and is often caused by an allergic reaction. One in five people will experience angioedema in their lifetime, with the swelling usually going within 24-72 hours. The GP may prescribe antihistamine medication recommended to help deal with the swelling.

Angioedema had appeared in one of my patients who had suffered from this condition for two years. She had lived in Spain for three years and, after a stressful return to the UK, she had developed a small wheal on her lip. It got worse and worse until she ended up in A&E several times and was finally referred to a dermatologist and treated with antihistamines.

Determined to get to the root of the problem, she kept a food diary but could find no pattern. To her knowledge she had never been allergic to anything in her life before. However, while in Spain her cat had become very ill with what the vet said was a parasitic infection, needing 30 days of treatment. She was responsible for cleaning the cat's litter tray during this time, but didn't fall ill. About a year later she had experienced severe sickness and diarrhoea, and later discovered, via a Quantum Bio Scan, that she had been subjected to 'an amoeba similar to Giardia'.

Angioedema has been linked to Giardia, as has urticaria [8] and atopic dermatitis,[9] so it is possible, in cases where a skin condition is not responding to treatment, and a digestive / bowel disorder is also present, that Giardia, or indeed other parasites, may be the hidden cause. Remember that Giardia can be present with no apparent underlying bowel symptoms.

Allergies can have a very debilitating affect on our health and by eradicating Giardia this can greatly improve the quality of life as in Maureen's case.

Maureen's story

Maureen had suffered a litany of allergy-linked problems for many years, which included eczema, a host of chemical sensitivities, reactions to foods, cats, petrol fumes, coal fires and many more. She had been seen in various clinics, in the UK and abroad, and had been prescribed a host of medicines including creams, pills, vitamin injections and steroids. Eventually Maureen came to me for treatment. She writes:

In 2010 I read an article in the Telegraph newspaper entitled: 'It hurt to even eat strawberries'. It was about the herbalist Susan Koten at the Willow Herbal Centre in Harold Wood. I made an appointment to see her and she diagnosed that I had Giardia lamblia, a parasite, and she put me on a course of wormwood for a week. It was truly a miracle. I could eat so many foods that I had been unable to eat for 30 years. I felt better than I had for a long time and stopped losing weight.

I still cannot eat certain foods and if I do by mistake I usually get a headache, which I can work through rather than retiring to bed. Maybe I will always have to be careful but I am so grateful to Susan for giving me my life back. I believe the doctors (most of them) did their best to help me but I think they only treated the symptoms and not the cause. One doctor, when I asked him what had caused the eczema, just said, 'Why does the sun come out and the moon shine?' and shrugged his shoulders.

Summary

A Giardia infestation can aggravate an established, pre-existing allergy, as the parasite will weaken an already overworked immune system. The immune system has to manufacture antibodies to deal with the invader and its cunning strategies of evasion, as discussed in Chapter 1. This further weakens the already compromised immune system, triggering an exacerbation of the infected person's allergy symptoms.

Giardia has an extraordinary ability to adapt to its surroundings, which enables it to survive and thrive very successfully whilst its host may be coughing and wheezing and experiencing chronic diarrhoea in a vain attempt to expel the Giardia from his/her body.

As we have seen in this chapter, giardiasis can result in consequences far beyond textbook gut problems. The next chapter looks at the implications of gallbladder involvement in Giardia infestation.

Chapter 8

The gallbladder connection

After observing patients for a number of years, I realised that just killing off Giardia in the stomach/small intestine area was not always sufficient and that something else was often needed. One patient in particular found that she felt fine while taking the wormwood I prescribed, but once she had finished the treatment, all her symptoms returned. On one occasion of muscle testing I identified her gallbladder as a problem and realised that I needed to flush this through with herbs as it seemed likely that trophozoites and/or cysts were infesting that organ. As soon as I started to follow this protocol her recovery became sustained.

The duodenum is where the trophozoites are released from their cyst form and where they then begin the process of producing more cysts in the presence of bile, for excretion into the faeces. The common bile duct, which runs from the gallbladder to the duodenum, allows bile to be excreted into the duodenum via the 'sphincter of Oddi', a muscular valve that controls the flow of digestive juices into the second part of the duodenum.

There have been reported cases of Giardia trophozoites and cysts being found in the gallbladder,[1] and I find in approximately 60% of my patients that the gallbladder is affected. It is my belief that trophozoites are able to travel into the common bile duct when the sphincter either opens up to release bile or is faulty, allowing trophozoites to cross over into the duct and travel to the gallbladder.

This may create a blockage, or partial blockage, and bile cannot be secreted efficiently. Without bile in the biliary tract pale-coloured fatty stools and jaundice may result due to fats not being digested properly. There may be some pain in the mid-upper or right-upper quadrant of the abdomen, with discomfort after eating fatty foods.

The role of the gallbladder

The gallbladder is a little pear-shaped sac which is located under the liver in the upper right-hand section of the abdomen and its job is to store the bile which is made by the liver. Bile is a combination of fluids, fat and cholesterol, and is designed specifically to help neutralise and break down fatty foods as they travel through the digestive system. When needed, bile is released into the duodenum (the first part of the small intestine) by the gallbladder, and helps the fat-soluble vitamins and nutrients to be more easily absorbed into the bloodstream by emulsifying the fats.

If Giardia has invaded the gallbladder then I give the patient a gallbladder tincture made up of various herbs, together with the *Artemisia annua* (sweet wormwood), to ensure the infestation is cleared from the body.

Gallbladder removal – cholecystectomy

Many people have had their gallbladders removed owing to the formation of stones inside the little sac. These stones are formed when there is too much cholesterol or bilirubin in the bile, or too little bile salt available, and the gallbladder is unable to empty as it should. I have often wondered if these stones could sometimes be caused by the body encasing the trophozoites to contain them?

A study carried out by the University of Edinburgh showed the removal of the gallbladder to be a very common operation, with about 60,000 procedures carried out each year.[2]

Gallbladder removal and Giardia

If a person has an infestation of Giardia, removing the gallbladder will not relieve the parasitic symptoms and it is only by eliminating giardiasis that relief will be achieved. As previously mentioned, the gallbladder is a storage sac for the bile produced by the liver. Removing the gallbladder causes bile delivery to become dysregulated, and as a result of this change, bile is continually released directly into the duodenum. In this circumstance, if Giardia are present, they will be constantly flooded with bile, which is a perfect situation for them to continue making new cysts.

This following case history is an example of how Giardia can take hold regardless of whether there is a gallbladder in situ or not. This patient, who I will call Carol, was experiencing bowel problems for years and having her gallbladder removed did not help.

Carol's story

Carol came to see me in 2010 with symptoms of irritable bowel syndrome (IBS), noisy intestines, bloating, gas and wind, alternating diarrhoea and constipation, constant nausea, bad breath and chronic fatigue. She had mucus in her stools, and these smelled offensive and varied in colour from yellow to brown. Her sleep was disturbed, and she was also suffering from shortness of breath and memory problems.

In May 2004, Carol had her gallbladder removed, along with around 100 yellowy green gallstones made up of hardened cholesterol; they looked like a handful of capers (see Figure 8.1).

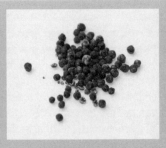

Figure 8.1: Gallstones removed from Carol's gallbladder

She had had stomach problems for 10 years before coming to me. In 2000 she had lost her grandmother and during that time she had suffered from a mixture of constipation and diarrhoea, which she put down to emotional distress. Following the loss, she had gone to Thailand for a month and said that following this trip her digestion had returned to a normal pattern for her.

In 2001 she got married and six months later fell pregnant with her first child. Tummy aches, wind and constipation continued to plague her. She gave me this account:

I thankfully sailed through my pregnancy but then ended up with a caesarean section as my baby was in the breach position.

Four months after my son had been born we moved house. I had had terrible chest pains for a while but put it down to stress with the move and a new baby to care for. A month after moving into our house, I collapsed and was taken to hospital. By this time, I was jaundiced too. I was diagnosed with gallstones. They flushed me through by inserting a catheter directly into my gallbladder to irrigate it with a form of ether to relieve the blocked stone to make the jaundice subside, but two months later the same thing happened again. I was then flushed through, and four months later had my gallbladder removed.

I returned to work not long after and continued to manage with the upset tummy and constant aches. I fell pregnant with my second child in 2005 and had the worst nine months ever. The only day I was not sick or suffering from an upset stomach was the day I went into labour. Again, I ended up with a caesarean section as my baby had 'got stuck'.

Things appeared to settle down for a while and when my daughter was 18 months old we moved house. Four months later I contracted pneumonia and pleurisy. After a week in hospital I was sent home to recuperate. I was constantly tired and this fatigue just did not seem to lift. Finally, after four months, I was given the all clear to return to work. I had reduced my hours to help combat the tiredness but it did not help, so after a few weeks I returned to my normal hours. I just had to get on with it.

As the years went by I was convinced it was just the way I was, continually tired and going from diarrhoea to constipation on a far too frequent basis. I had mentioned it to the nurse when I went for a birth control check up and she just said it sounded hormonal. The fact it was not a regular pattern unlike my monthly periods seemed a bit strange to me, but what else could I do? I had explained that if it was a good day I was a whole dress size different to when it was a 'bad' day. Also, that the pain started as a griping pain just under my ribs but by the time it reached the bottom of my tummy it was like labour pains – totally horrendous! Then came the explosiveness of needing a bathroom – there and then. I had tried cutting out foods that I thought were upsetting me – fresh bread, red meat - but it made little difference.

Then from Christmas of 2010 I started to feel sick; sometimes it would last all day; other days it was just in the morning. By April it had got to the point that it would last all day, every day, and I had developed a pain in my ribs – it felt like when I was pregnant with a foot wedged in my ribs – only I was not pregnant.

I went to the doctor. First, he prescribed some antacid tablets as he thought I might have a stomach ulcer, but that did not explain the pain in my ribs. My daily bowel habit was awful – I was always full of wind and suffering more and more from diarrhoea. It was giving me no warning, and when I had to go I had to go; it was just awful.

They sent me for an ultrasound scan, which showed nothing. I then had a colonoscopy and again this did not show anything so the consultant said the problem was 'irritable bowel.'

Having felt so ill for so long, Carol decided to go for an allergy test at her local health shop, and was advised to avoid sodium bicarbonate, the grape family of fruits, food additives E334 and E335 (as used in fizzy drinks, jams, jellies etc), E336 mono-potassium L-tartrate (as used in wine and packet lemon pie mix), E336 di potassium L-tartrate (as used in the jelly part of packet trifle mix), E337 potassium sodium L-tartrate (as used in meat and cheese products), and also tea, honey and plums.

She was drinking a lot of fizzy drinks and cordials but noticed some improvement in her condition when, on the advice of the practitioner at her local health shop, she gave these up.

When she picked up her allergy tests, she was given an article about me and my treatment of parasites. She told me:

As I read it, it was like someone else had written about my life for the last 10 years or so!

On her first visit to my clinic I diagnosed a Giardia infestation and I also found the energies through her kidneys and thyroid were weak. On checking her pulse, I could not feel any pulsation at any point along the surface radial artery on each wrist. The pulse should feel strong and firm under my fingertips, with a good regular beat. When I cannot feel a pulse, it could be because the person is holding onto fluid and that their kidney energy is weak and unable to clear fluids from their body efficiently; this was the case with Carol. The kidney energy field is the powerhouse of the body so this tied in with the overall poor energy levels which Carol was experiencing.

I gave her wormwood, and told her to take two teaspoons three times a day to kill off the Giardia parasite. I also gave her a 'kidney mix', and a tincture for her thyroid.

She didn't find the herbs pleasant tasting but was determined to stick with them. After two days she felt brighter, and her husband said she was less restless when she was asleep. She told me:

I felt human! Four days later, the mixture tasted totally different and something had definitely changed.

Even Carol's friends and family noticed how much brighter she looked. Three weeks on, she told me:

I have had so much more energy and in fact I have not needed my afternoon 'siesta' once since treatment started. I have been able to do so much more and I have not needed to locate a toilet with any hurry – it has improved my confidence and also added to what we can and cannot do as a family. Days out as just mum and two kids were being put on hold if I was having a 'bad' day as I could not leave them outside the toilet or take them in with me. Now we can go anywhere.

In over 60% of the patients I see with a Giardia infestation, the gallbladder is affected, and by definition, the digestive health of the patient. With over 60,000 cholecystectomies performed each year by the NHS, and the wide prevalence of giardiasis, it would seem sensible, in my opinion, and as part of the diagnostic process, for health professionals to eliminate the possibility of a Giardia infestation before the surgical option is taken.

Gallbladder checklist

For anyone facing surgery to remove their gallbladder, it might be prudent to consider the following questions prior to booking the operation. Do you suffer from any of the following symptoms on a regular basis:
1. loose stools that are pale yellow/putty coloured?
2. difficulty in digesting fatty foods?
3. discomfort after eating fatty foods?
4. pain in your right shoulder blade?
5. pain in the mid/right upper quadrant of your abdomen?
6. nausea/vomiting?
7. noisy intestines?
8. bloating?
9. gas/wind?

10. fatigue?
11. loss of sleep?
12. fever and chills?

If the answer is 'yes' to six or more of these symptoms, then I recommend eliminating the possibility of a Giardia infestation by seeking an ELISA stool test to ensure giardiasis is not the cause of the problems.

Summary

Treating the gallbladder and getting rid of the Giardia trophozoites and/or cysts can make all the difference to successfully eradicating this parasite. The trophozoites congregate around the bile duct because this alkaline environment is important for their transformation into cysts, which are then egested in the faeces ready to infect the next host. The gallbladder can become diseased from this invasion and this is a possible cause for removal of this organ being recommended.

The pancreas is positioned close to the gallbladder and Giardia may also create havoc within that organ. Its impact on insulin production and the health issues that arise from that are explained in the next chapter.

Chapter 9

The pancreas connection

In the last chapter we saw how key the gallbladder is in a Giardia infestation. This also links Giardia to diabetes, because the gallbladder and pancreas share the same drainage duct into the small intestine.

So, let's just take a look at diabetes and what a growing problem it is. The National Health Service (NHS) currently spends almost 10% of its entire budget treating the repercussions of type 2 diabetes, while further millions of pounds are being poured into the quest for finding a cure. Coffee,[1] barley,[2] and even Viagra,[3] have all (subject to further research) been touted as potential aids to lowering the risk of getting type 2 diabetes in recent years and, with around three million type 2 diabetics and a further 11.9 million people at risk of the condition in the UK alone, such apparently simple solutions are, not surprisingly, music to our ears. We'd all love to think there's a cure just around the corner, and preferably one we can access easily.

There are two distinct types of diabetes but the problems associated with them are similar. Type 1 occurs when the body is unable to produce insulin. About 10% of people with diabetes have type 1. No one knows exactly what causes it, and it usually affects children or young adults, starting suddenly and getting worse quickly. Treated with daily insulin doses, taken either by injection or via an insulin pump, a child diagnosed with type 1 at the age of five faces up to 19,000 injections and 50,000 finger pricks by the time they are 18 according to the Juvenile Diabetes Research Foundation.[4]

More is known about type 2 diabetes, particularly relating to risk factors; in type 2, although the body can still produce and regulate insulin, its ability to do so is impaired. Risk factors that contribute to this disease include family history, age and being overweight. Obesity, especially around the abdomen, is thought to trigger changes to the body's metabolism due to the build-up of fat around the vital organs. This includes the pancreas, the organ that produces insulin. These changes can then affect how the cells in the body use the insulin produced by beta cells in the pancreas, leading to 'insulin resistance'. This means cells in the body become unresponsive to insulin and are unable to use it effectively. The combination of insulin resistance and ineffective use causes glucose (sugar) to build up in the blood, leading to type 2 diabetes. However, there is a lot of overlap between type 1 and type 2. People can have features of both, and both types are on the increase.

So, what is the link with Giardia? It is all to do with the anatomy of our digestive organs.

The duodenum is the first part of the small intestine. It is where pancreatic enzymes and bile are introduced to aid in digestion, and these enzymes need an alkaline environment in order to function properly. It is exactly the kind of alkaline environment in which the trophozoites, hatched from the Giardia cysts, can thrive, and in cases of infection there will be an abundance of them congregating around the pancreatic duct where it joins the bile duct (attached to the gallbladder) to open into the duodenum. The Giardia love the alkaline environment, and the salts in the bile at this point encourage the production of new cysts. The trophozoites and cysts can easily slip into the bile or pancreatic ducts and cause problems with the functioning of the gallbladder and/or the pancreas. Giardia in the pancreas can also interfere with insulin levels.

Understanding the pancreas

The pancreas is both an endocrine (ductless) and exocrine (with a duct) gland. The endocrine part secretes two hormones which regulate blood sugar levels – insulin, from the beta cells, and glucagon, from the alpha cells. Insulin tends to decrease blood glucose levels, while glucagon increases them. In other words, glucagon and insulin have antagonistic effects, with glucagon promoting the production of glucose and releasing it into the bloodstream, and insulin helping to move glucose into cells from the bloodstream while also inhibiting its removal from storage as glycogen

Unhealthy diets have a lot to do with pancreatic problems. Eating too many sugary foods, such as sweets, biscuits, cakes, and even pastas and breads, can cause an overload of sugar in the body. This creates blood sugar imbalances that can lead to diseases like diabetes.

Maintaining a healthy pancreas

Introducing a healthy eating regime is one way of maintaining a healthy pancreas. Foods such as omega-3-rich fish, nuts, vegetables, beans and fruit will help to protect against pancreatic diseases as will eating raw and unprocessed foods when possible.[4]

For anyone suffering from diabetes and for those who just want to lose weight, the Rainbow diet is certainly worth considering. The kaleidoscope of colourful foods in this Mediterranean diet will not only help to reduce weight and symptoms for type 2 diabetics, but has the added benefit of lowering the risk of developing any cancer.[5]

It's also important to keep stress under control if possible, as stress has been implicated as a trigger for the onset of diabetes in people who are already predisposed to developing the disease.

Chapter 9

Stress hormones in the body can have a deleterious effect on glycaemic (blood sugar) control and can be a major problem for effective glucose control. Helping to relieve stress is shown to keep diabetes under control.[6] In my opinion, a Giardia infestation should also be investigated as a background factor in diabetes. To illustrate this point, I would like to share the story of a young patient of mine, called Alice.

Alice's story

Alice came into my clinic with her mother on 1 October 2010 with a history of type 1 diabetes. They were in a desperate situation as Alice had been admitted to hospital nine times over the previous two years and had had numerous consultations with three diabetic specialists and yet her diabetes was still totally out of control and threatening her life. Alice had, for some reason, become resistant to insulin.

The presenting symptoms on her first visit were fatigue, headache, anger, sickness, stomach cramps, cold extremities, disturbed sleep, dizziness, alternating stool patterns, offensive smelling stools, wind and bloating. Could Giardia be the cause of Alice's insulin resistance? This is her experience, which became a featured article in the magazine What Doctors Don't Tell You (January 2013 edition).

Alice had been diagnosed as a type 1 diabetic at the age of 9 years and had had to inject insulin into her body daily. This had controlled her condition until 2008. On a school trip to India that summer her insulin had become exposed to the heat and lost its effectiveness, or so Alice had thought at the time; she had become very unwell and ended up in hospital in Leh, India. Alice, now in her final year at secondary school, began to have much higher blood sugar readings without any change to her diet or lifestyle.

After completing her A levels in 2009, Alice had numerous contacts with the diabetic team at her local hospital as she was unable to keep her blood sugar levels down with her usual injections of insulin. Their advice was to keep increasing her meal-time insulin dose from 6 to 30 units of Novorapid with food, but this still did not achieve control.

After a holiday to France with her family, where she was again admitted to hospital with high sugar levels, Alice consulted another doctor privately.

Alice said:

He changed my medication so I could split the dose with injections, one in the morning and one in the evening, and advised that I increase my meal-time doses. This doctor said 'insulin works', basically doubting my compliance. I was now injecting 120 units per day and 10 days before I was due to start at Leeds University I was admitted to hospital to be 'rebalanced'. I was put on an intravenous drip and my blood sugar levels became more normal.

At Leeds University I started to study for a BSc in Clinical physiology/cardiology but my condition still continued to deteriorate and in October 2009 I went to A&E as I felt very unwell and dizzy, but after five hours I was discharged without my blood sugar levels/ketones being tested. That night and throughout the following day I was continuously vomiting and I was admitted to hospital with diabetic ketoacidosis.

In May 2010 I was put on an insulin pump and, although the pump made it easier to have such large doses of insulin, my sugar levels stayed high and I was again admitted to hospital. I was now no longer able to continue my studies and returned home to Beaconsfield, Buckinghamshire. My doctor at my local hospital did little to help me, suggesting my problem was due to the incorrect use of the pump. He treated me as if I was the problem and was extremely dismissive when my parents suggested that something else could be the cause of the problem. The phrase we kept hearing was 'insulin works', which clearly it didn't.

We went privately to see another doctor at the London Medical Centre, who changed my insulin back to the old-style Actrapid, but that made no difference.

I returned to Leeds at the beginning of September to get on with my life but it soon became apparent that I could not do so. The doctor at the London Medical Centre suggested a hospital admission so that he could assess what was happening with my absorption of the insulin.

In the meantime, my mother read an article in the Daily Telegraph about a woman who had suffered from severe stomach problems for 40 years. She had been to Susan Koten at the Willow Herbal Centre in Harold Wood, Essex, who had diagnosed a parasite called Giardia and prescribed a herbal remedy which consisted of wormwood. My mother was beginning to wonder if perhaps I had picked up Giardia on my trip to India in 2008 as it was at this time that I had developed insulin resistance. In sheer desperation my mother made an appointment for me to see Susan.

Susan diagnosed that I did have the parasite Giardia and she gave me the wormwood herbal medicine. Within days of taking the medicine my insulin resistance began to reduce. I took this medicine for two weeks, by which time the parasite had disappeared. My basal insulin requirements began to fall and correction doses started to work. I have been taking other herbal medicine prescribed by Susan since the middle of October 2010. Since then my basal rate has dropped from an average of 100 units a day (often increased by 150%) to 13 units currently.

I believe this dramatic turnaround can only be a result of the killing off of the parasite and the strengthening of my organs with herbal medicine. Although my health has improved and my diabetes returned to 'normal' this experience has completely overwhelmed me both physically and emotionally.

Alice is a qualified teacher who has her diabetes well under control and is leading a full, active and happy life.

I recently heard from Alice again (February 2019) and this is an excerpt from her correspondence.

I feel at peace. I feel happy, healthy and safe knowing that I found you and you helped me through such a terrible time. My diabetes is a lot more controlled now and I work hard every day to keep that going. As much of an awful experience that all was, it has put the most important thing at the foremost of my brain – 'health'. There is not a day that goes by that I am not grateful and appreciative of what I have and how I choose to live my life. My insulin requirements still vary depending on my life situations but I am able to control my blood sugar levels again. Thank you.

Alice's story seems extreme but she believes she would not have survived had she not taken the herbal route to identify and get rid of a Giardia infestation. Her story, and the one below, demonstrate how intrepid and persistent this tiny organism can be and how easily it can be missed (or not even looked for) when a person is already dealing with a complex and serious illness such as diabetes.

After I treated Alice, I was contacted by another young woman I will call Melanie who, at 27 years old, was also coming to terms with a diagnosis of type 1 diabetes. This is her story.

Melanie's story

I was diagnosed with the auto-immune disease type 1 diabetes in June 2017, at 27 years old. The diagnosis came as a complete shock and initially it was difficult to make the necessary changes to my life to stay healthy. I was told by doctors that I was in the 'honeymoon phase' which meant my pancreas was still producing some of its own insulin, so I only required two units of insulin twice a day. I am informed that at some point the honeymoon phase will end, my pancreas will stop making any insulin of its own and I will be taking a much higher volume of insulin each day to stay alive.

I am very lucky to have a supportive family and boyfriend who are helping me navigate this disease. My boyfriend, Ollie, spends a lot of time researching type 1 diabetes and one day came across an article in What Doctors Don't Tell You *discussing how Susan Koten had helped another girl with type 1 diabetes dramatically improve her health through the removal of parasites. This was the first connection I had come across that referenced both an auto-immune disease and parasites. On further research, I realised I was experiencing several symptoms that are present with parasite infections and have been for quite a few years, such as bloating, nausea, a weak immune system and fatigue. I had come to know these as 'normal' and until now had accepted them.*

After about six months of numerous doctors' appointments, where I was told that the only way to manage type 1 diabetes was to wait for the health of my pancreas to decline and to gradually increase my insulin injections, I was growing frustrated. Whilst I recognise there is currently no cure for this disease, I felt certain there must be something I could do to help support my pancreas. I wanted to search for the cause of what could have triggered the auto immune response in my body to attack the insulin-creating cells in my pancreas, and to find out whether I could heal that root problem, in the hope of slowing or stopping further damage. It felt like a long shot, but I had to try, and the article that Ollie had come across a while ago filled me with hope. I decided to visit Susan to see if she could help me.

At my appointment with Susan she asked me to hold out my arm, applied gentle pressure on my wrist with one hand, while hovering the other hand over different parts of my body. I found I could easily hold my arm in place with little effort, until she held her hand over my pancreas and then my stomach. In both instances my arm waivered and dropped, as though I had no muscles in my arm, despite the incredibly light pressure being applied. Susan then took out a box of small containers that held different parasites within them. Using the same technique, holding her hand over the containers, she was able to decipher which parasites I had by the response from my left arm. She confirmed that I had three parasites, one of which was Giardia, and they were in both my pancreas and my gut. Aside from this, Susan noticed other issues that were contributing to my current state of health, both physically and mentally, which she helped me to resolve there and then. For example, she used the gentle and pain-free Bowen technique to correct my misaligned hip and jaw. I was given a couple of tonics to take for a week, three times a day, to remove the parasites from my system. The process was non-intrusive and gentle, as the parasites passed unknowingly through my stools. I was also given herbal sprays to improve the health of my pancreas, immune system and thyroid. I booked a follow-up appointment for a week's time to review my progress. I left feeling like a weight had been lifted and extremely grateful to have met Susan.

I visited Susan twice more and by the third visit it was happily confirmed that my body was clear of all parasites. I could feel the difference in my body as my energy had returned, I wasn't bloated after meals, I stopped feeling nauseous and I was no longer hungry all the time. I only needed to use the immune system and thyroid herbal spray for a week, however I am currently using the pancreas spray as an ongoing measure. The sprays are such a simple and easy way of improving my health it felt too good to be true, however I could feel such a difference in my body. Being recently diagnosed, I am seeing a slight increase in the amount of insulin I need to inject as time progresses. However, a year later I am only taking three units of insulin twice a day, which I am told is incredible. Doctors have been amazed and surprised that I'm on such a small amount and that I'm doing so well. I contribute a large part of this to the removal of parasites from my body which were compromising my immune system and the capacity of my pancreas, the pancreas herbal spray, and a healthy low-carbohydrate and low-sugar diet. I have noticed on the occasion that I forget to use the pancreas spray my blood glucose levels increase, then return to a balanced level as soon as I resume use, which clearly shows me that it's helping maintain the health of my pancreas. Being diagnosed with Type 1 Diabetes left me feeling vulnerable and as though I didn't have control of my future. Receiving healing and guidance from Susan, along with the support of those close to me, has helped me regain confidence and hope for the future. My appointments with Susan completely changed my outlook and the way that I take care of my body, on every level.

By including Alice's and Melanie's stories, I hope to alert readers, particularly those who are insulin resistant, to the possibility that Giardia infestation might be the cause when their 'normal' symptoms start to behave differently.

Summary

The pancreas is another important organ that can be invaded and disrupted by the presence of Giardia; the consequences can even be life threatening.

The next chapter looks at how to prevent this very prolific and unwelcome guest from entering our bodies and taking over our lives, in a very disruptive and debilitating manner.

Chapter 10

Prevention

When one of my patients asked her GP about Giardia, the 60-year-old doctor said he had seen only one case, despite having been practising as a medic since his 20s. To me, that confession is quite astounding when you only have to look at the lifecycle of this parasite to see how easily it can be transmitted. All it needs is for someone who is already infected to fail to wash their hands thoroughly, and the parasite can be pretty sure of quickly finding its way into someone else and setting up home. It can be passed from animals to humans, and from one family member to another, within hours.

However, not everyone who comes into contact with it is infected as a result. The environment Giardia requires is specific, as already discussed in previous chapters, and has to be right for Giardia to establish itself and flourish. In some people, it will be destroyed and eliminated by the immune system's defence mechanism. I have treated a family of two adults and two children who all seemed to have come into contact with Giardia from their grandfather. The mother and daughter had become infected and the father and son remained well. So why was this? The reason is not obvious but, in my experience, I have noticed the less anxious someone is in their general demeanour, the less likely they are to become infected. It does not apply in every case, but we have already discussed how stress can negatively affect the immune system, so this observation, for me, reinforces the importance of maintaining a healthy gut microbiome (see Chapter 6), especially when faced with the challenges an infestation of Giardia can create.

Here are some of the more common routes of transmission:

- **Dirty water** – My plumber called me one day complaining of stomach pains. He told me he was repairing a radiator and to get the water to flow he had sucked on the pipe and got a mouthful of stagnant water. He subsequently developed severe stomach pains. I diagnosed giardiasis and he responded very quickly to the herbal protocol (see Chapter 11). So, apart from avoiding swallowing water from old pipes, it is also advisable to avoid taking in water when swimming or playing in lakes, rivers, springs, ponds and streams where Giardia may live. Episodes of giardiasis have also been linked to public swimming pools, and Giardia is notoriously resistant to chlorine.[1] It only takes an infected child to defecate in a pool for the water to become a source of transmission.[2]

- **Public water coolers** – I was made aware of this problem by one of my patients, who worked in a bank. Mary had had severe digestive issues for about five years when she came to see me. I diagnosed she was suffering from giardiasis and gave her the wormwood tincture. This helped while she was taking it, but her digestive issues soon returned after she had completed the prescribed course. We looked at what she was eating and where she was eating and we could not see a clear link to her getting re-infected, yet her digestive issues continued as she kept repeatedly picking up the parasite. We then decided to look at the water she was drinking at work and she informed me she was getting her supply from a water cooler machine. She brought some to my clinic

and when we muscle-tested (see Chapter 2) the sample
of water, it showed there was a problem. Mary then
stopped drinking the water at work and used bottled
water instead. Her symptoms improved dramatically.
She also reported the incident to her company, who then
supplied her with bottled water.

- **Dirty surfaces** – We need to be aware that the parasite
  can live for months in its cyst form outside a host. If a
  person has a Giardia infestation and is suffering from
  diarrhoea, it is possible that whilst cleaning themselves
  with toilet paper, their hands can become soiled and,
  if they do not wash their hands thoroughly before
  leaving the bathroom, they can contaminate handles
  and surfaces, ensuring the next person to use the toilet
  facility will be exposed to infection.
- **Nappies** – Changing babies' nappies, or just carrying
  a young child whose dirty nappy leaks and gets onto
  hands, carries the same risks. Toys could also contain
  contaminated stool from an infected person or animal.
- **Close contact** – If one family member has contracted
  Giardia and brought it into the household, it can then
  be passed on to other family members. The person who
  is preparing the food needs to make sure they wash
  their hands thoroughly, especially if they might be a
  Giardia carrier. To deal with a Giardia infestation in
  a household, it is advisable for all family members to
  be tested and, if they are found to be positive carriers,
  also treated. I would not recommend treating just
  one member of the family without knowing who else
  has been infected as the risk of re-infection is great.
  Remember, if Giardia is in the family, and friends and
  relatives are staying, then there is a risk the infection
  may be passed onto them. Likewise, when visiting
  friends and/or family, eating and drinking at their

house, there is the possibility of contracting the parasite if they have Giardia symptoms.

- **Ice** – Avoid drinking iced water if there is uncertainty about where the water used to make the ice came from. The Centres for Disease Control and Prevention (CDC) advise not to use ice in developing countries as it is probably made from tap water,[3] so refusing ice in drinks is a good idea. If water is thought to be infected it needs to be boiled for at least one minute to kill off Giardia.
- **Public buildings** – Being where groups of people congregate and share food and drink creates a risk of infection.
- **Raw or partially cooked food** – We are all being encouraged to eat salads and raw vegetables, but we could be at risk if the food has become infected with unhealthy organisms during its preparation. It is vital to avoid anything that has not been thoroughly cooked to kill off parasites. All foods that are going to be eaten raw should be thoroughly washed in uncontaminated, preferably boiled, water.
- **Farm animals** – Giardia infections have been reported in sheep, cows (especially dairy calves), horses, pigs and goats, and could easily be passed on to those who work with animals, or those who visit 'petting' farms. Again, employing basic hygiene practices will ensure these prolific little parasites do not get a foothold in an unsuspecting visitor.
- **Pets** – Looking after our pets and our interaction with them is another activity where we are at risk of infection. We all love our animals and most treat them as members of the family; I certainly do. However, unless we are aware of the dangers we face by not practising good hygiene, we put ourselves and our families at risk. When

cleaning up after pets we must make sure our hands are thoroughly washed, including scrubbing under our nails or, better still, wear disposable gloves to avoid Giardia infection. Anal licking is a popular activity for dogs and if the dog has Giardia the cysts will be excreted in the faeces which may be passed on to the owner if the dog is allowed to lick around the owner's mouth. We don't like to think our dogs would do disgusting things like drinking from toilets if the opportunity arose but they do and if a dog drinks from a toilet which has been used by someone who has excreted Giardia cysts, the dog can become infected. The dog is equally at risk of picking up the parasite and bringing it into the home after rolling on the ground in fox faeces. One of my patients reported that she saw her cat drinking water from her glass by her bedside, and she felt this was the root of her infection.

- **Sexual activity** – Giardiasis does not need a large dose of Giardia cysts to infect its host. When cleaning ourselves after going to the toilet, somewhere in the region of 10-100 cysts can easily be moved from the anus across the perineum to the genitals. If sexual activity includes oral contact, then these cysts can be ingested by the unsuspecting partner, causing him or her to become infected.

Proton pump inhibitors

People who regularly take proton pump inhibitors (PPIs), such as omeprazole, to reduce their stomach acidity, may be more at risk of picking up a Giardia infestation than those who do not. PPIs work by blocking proteins in specialised cells within the stomach lining that pump acid into the stomach. This action reduces acid production, and having low stomach acid can not only give rise to symptoms of bloating, belching or flatulence after meals, but Giardia prefer a more alkaline environment and, therefore, are able to colonise and flourish in these conditions. Stomach acid helps the body break down protein and absorb important vitamins and minerals such as B12, calcium, iron and magnesium; it is also essential for killing harmful bacteria and parasites. Suppressing stomach acidity will decrease nutrient absorption, thereby weakening the immune system and allowing parasites like Giardia to breed.

Christopher's story

I found Susan Koten by chance and I'm sure glad I did. Having read some literature on the types of treatments offered at the Willow Herbal Centre, I decided to ring and make an appointment. My symptoms were primarily to do with digestive problems associated with IBS, which I had suffered from for many years. I also suffered from acid reflux and was taking a PPI called Losec [a brand of omeprazole] to help me cope with this.

As with many people who suffer from IBS, I had tried various things to improve the condition in terms of dietary changes but without much success.

During my initial consultation with Susan, I explained my symptoms, and mentioned as well as IBS that I also suffered from bad headaches and was taking paracetamol every day to try and deal with them. This had been going on for months.

Susan diagnosed the Giardia parasite as the cause of my IBS symptoms and I was prescribed two herbal treatments. Over the course of the following week my digestive system settled down, my stomach felt great and for the first time in years I did not have any of the symptoms associated with IBS. Also, the headaches which had been constant each day were now completely gone. I had almost forgotten what it felt like to be headache free and not to have to take painkillers each day.

Christopher's job meant he travelled a great deal and he seemed prone to picking up the parasite. He would frequently update me on his ups and downs with Giardia, and when he was in England I would prescribe a course of my herbal remedy to deal with the parasite. On one such visit Christopher told me:

Not having Giardia generally means I do not have any symptoms at all and can lead a 'normal life'.

Christopher decided he would stop taking the PPI which he'd been taking for his acid reflux problems. He was aware the Giardia parasite preferred an alkaline environment and he wanted to see if a higher level of acidity in his stomach would create a healthier digestive system and prevent him from attracting Giardia so frequently.

A short time later, Christopher wrote:

It's been 2½ weeks since I stopped taking the Losec (omeprazole) and things are going okay. Very little acid reflux to mention and just occasionally feel nauseous. I just take a piece of ginger (soaked in hot water) and the feeling goes away. Also, no symptoms of the parasite to report and long may it last. I'm still being very sensible with my diet and making sure that I eat the right things. If I do decide to treat myself, it's only in small doses.

Understanding the risk

We all like to think we are scrupulous in our hygiene habits, and that the surfaces we regularly come into contact with do not present a danger to us, but research from the London School of Hygiene and Tropical Medicine, and Queen Mary, University of London,[4] found that one in six mobile phones is contaminated with faecal matter, with the most likely reason being that people do not adequately wash their hands, not only after using the toilet, but at any time.

The facts discovered in this study are quite shocking and reinforce the need for all of us to be vigilant in our hand washing hygiene, both in and outside our home environment. It is also important to teach children the importance of washing their hands, with soap, whenever they have been exposed to possible infection. It must become a habit for us all if we are to avoid not only Giardia infection, but all the other possible contaminants we are exposed to every day.

The World Health Organization is fully aware of the role good hand hygiene plays in the containment of infectious diseases and how important it is that we follow their guidelines and pass this important message on to our children. They have addressed this in many ways over the years and I have referenced their directive on hand hygiene for those interested in this topic.[5] In my view, if this protocol were more widely known and adhered to by the general population, problems like Giardia infestations would decrease.

How does Giardia get into drinking water?

Millions of Giardia parasites can be released in one bowel movement of an infected human, or animal, and this waste can enter municipal drinking water systems through a number of different routes. This can include sewage overflows, sewage systems that are not working properly, polluted storm water run-off and agricultural run-off. Wells may be more vulnerable to such contamination after flooding, particularly if they are shallow, have been dug or bored, or have been submerged by floodwater for long periods of time.

What about *my* drinking water?

Many people obtain their drinking water from private wells and for those living in England and Wales who are concerned their water may be contaminated, the Drinking Water Inspectorate (DWI) was formed in 1990 to provide independent reassurance that water supplies in England and Wales were safe and drinking water quality was acceptable to consumers. If contacted, they will supply a list of laboratories by area that will perform tests on drinking water for a fee.

How can Giardia be removed from drinking water?

An effective way to kill or inactivate Giardia in drinking water, is to boil the water for at least one minute; this will ensure any contamination is swiftly dealt with. Home water filters are another way of dealing with the problem and filters using the reverse osmosis method will do the trick. There are also many ultraviolet systems on the market which can eliminate organisms and harmful bacteria from well water. However, not all filters remove parasites so it is always best to check before purchasing a filter. Alternatively, and again, if you are in the UK, look for a filter carrying the National Sanitation Federation (NSF) Standard 53.

How can giardiasis be prevented?

Anyone who has ever been affected by Giardia will want to know how to prevent a re-infestation, but the following advice should apply to us all:

- **Be water wary:** Giardia is a water-borne parasite and any accidental consumption of unclean water is a risk, especially when travelling. It is important, if you are concerned about the water supply, to drink only bottled water that's been sold in a sealed and tamper-proof bottle from a known manufacturer. Water from an unknown source should be purified by boiling for at least one minute, especially if it is to be used for cleaning teeth. Chemical purification tablets are a good back-up if boiled water is not available, but it should be noted they are not as reliable, and can also make the water taste foul. Avoid salads and fruit that may have been washed in unsafe water.
- **Wash hands thoroughly:** As referenced earlier, this

is a must, especially before and after eating food, and most especially after using the toilet. The World Health Organization recommends we wash our hands for as long as it takes to sing two full rounds of *Happy Birthday To You!* Soap should always be used.

- **Laundry:** Giardia cysts cannot survive for longer than 10 minutes in a water temperature of 54° Celsius (130°F) or higher. The Centers for Disease Control (CDC) in the US advise that the clothing of infected people, and some pet items such as bedding and cloth toys, should be washed at temperatures high enough to kill off the parasite, and then heat-dried at the highest temperature for 30 minutes. This practice should continue while a person or pet in the home has a Giardia infection.[6]
- **Red clover as a preventative:** I have started to use *Trifolium pratense* (red clover) as a preventative herb. This has the ability to stop Giardia trophozoites from latching onto the intestinal wall and, therefore, can keep re-infection at bay – see Appendix I (page 129) for more information.
- **Keep candida in check:** Infection with the yeast *Candida albicans* can often go hand in hand with a Giardia infestation and may be an underlying digestive issue for many years following infection. Giardia infestation can weaken the immune system and Candida can then easily become established, often giving rise to digestive symptoms similar to Giardia.
- **Love your 'bugs':** Maintaining a healthy bacterial environment in the gut can help to keep Giardia at bay and seems to be one reason why two people who eat the same food and live in the same environment can respond completely differently to contact with the parasite. One may not suffer any consequences, while the other may become extremely ill. We see the same

difference in response to bacterial gastrointestinal infections too. One may be protected by their probiotic flora, while the other, whose microbiome is depleted, may be less fortunate. Antibiotics, poor diet (especially one that is high in sugar) and compromised immunity can adversely affect gut flora. The contraceptive pill, prolonged stress, dentistry work and exposure to toxic substances can also adversely affect the gut flora. Disruptions to the balance of probiotics in the gut can compromise the beneficial roles they play in the body, and people with an imbalance between probiotics and pathogens may experience poor digestion, lowered natural immunity and a large variety of conditions such as:

o   low energy levels
o   poor immunity
o   gas or bloating
o   food intolerances or allergies
o   acne and/or eczema
o   indigestion, heartburn
o   constipation or diarrhoea
o   thrush and/or candida overgrowth
o   Irritable Bowel Syndrome (IBS)
o   Inflammatory Bowel Disease (IBD).

- **Look after your immune system:** This cannot be over emphasised; we saw the importance of this in Chapter 6.

An undetected visitor like Giardia does not only negatively affect the general health of the host, and make life thoroughly miserable the longer it goes on, but it can also have a significant impact on the bank balance as sufferers search for answers and relief from its debilitating effects.

Chapter 10

Tony's story

I went on holiday to Kenya six years ago and wanted to rally with the locals in each and every way; the best opportunity was in the eating joints. Friends and relatives took me to eat out in various places. I sampled roadside food, I ate in houses that had no fridge or even electricity, I ate in five-star hotels. During that holiday I stayed in a house that belonged to a well-to-do family, even by western standards, but as I now know I could have picked up pathogens in that house too.

Problems really started during that two-week holiday. I started off with what I thought was travellers' diarrhoea, which was on and off. When I came back to the UK I bought the most expensive probiotic I could find in the hope that my bowel would return to normal. I then started bloating and getting cramps. The diarrhoea stopped but the bloating and the cramps intensified. I could not empty my bowels properly and at night I felt the food I had eaten earlier was sitting just below my throat. In the meantime, I had radically changed my diet – no sugar, no dairy of any sort, no wheat, no red meat, no caffeine. As I do not drink alcohol I did not have any difficulty with that aspect of my new lifestyle.

I spent many hours online daily looking for answers and buying anything that promised to address the situation I was in. I bought parasite cleansers, vitamins, a £300 water distiller, an ozone air-purifier as I thought fresh air would make my nights bearable. I sent my stool sample to a lab that was recommended a lot by the online community, but the results were all negative. Over the past six years I have spent nearly £10,000 on health products and services. Throughout all this my GP was trying the best he could to help, but every test that he did came back negative.

I tried MMS (Miracle Mineral Supplement), I tried ozonated olive oil, I tried tinctures of all kinds and in different combinations, olive leaf extract, horsetail, wormwood, clove, garlic tablets, mastic gum – the list is endless. I used Epsom salts at least twice a week on bad weeks and sometimes castor oil so that I could empty my bowels fully. In the meantime, the smell coming from my stomach was revolting even to myself. I knew I had really bad breath the moment I started to talk even without capping my mouth. I could not stand my own body odour – my sweat smelt really bad, I could fill up a large room with sulphur-smelling gas within a minute of two, my digestive system was acting like a bio-gas production chamber.

I may have successfully treated myself many times over with the various things I was taking, but I always got re-infected and assumed I had not cleared the pathogens.

As I was Googling my symptoms I came across an article online talking about the parasite Giardia and how some herbs had been used to treat the person affected. I was excited and looked up the herbalist who happened to be Susan Koten. I rang and was able to get an appointment for myself and my whole family.

The key to my health was the revelation that I had to have the whole family clear of the pathogens in order for me to be totally cured. As only my wife handles my food she was the main person to target for the treatment besides me. It is now two weeks since I finished the herbal dose I was given and I have continued to improve daily; I have even started to visit people who I could not visit because of the bad breath issue. I can eat anything I want without any bloating thereafter. I can now say life is good. Susan gave me my life back, and in the process saved me the thousands of pounds I was spending every year trying to get better.

Summary

The Giardia parasite cannot be seen with the naked eye and, therefore, most of us are blissfully unaware of its existence. It is only when we experience ill health that we may become aquainted with it, but the importance of good personal hygiene practices are key if we want to lower our risk of infection.

For those unfortunate enough to become infected with this resilient little parasite, the next chapter deals with the treatment protocol.

Chapter 11

Treating giardiasis

So, what do we know about Giardia? Well, it has been living with us for many years, and has learned to adapt very successfully to its surroundings. We also know we do not have to be travelling abroad to pick it up, it is quite happily living among us wherever we are, using our bodies to continue its breeding activities. It is rarely looked for as a cause of 'belly' related problems and we are frequently told its effects (giardiasis) are irritable bowel syndrome (IBS). We need to be aware that it is more common than we are generally led to believe.

A Giardia infection is one of the most common causes of water-borne disease in the United States, according to the Mayo Clinic.[1] There is no drug or vaccine available to prevent infection, and the only advice on prevention from the medical professionals is to take a 'common sense' approach regarding hygiene, as we have discussed earlier (see Chapter 10).

For those patients lucky enough to get an early diagnosis from their doctor, a variety of antibiotic medications is available to kill off the parasite, and in many cases, a single course of the chosen drug will be sufficient to deal with the invader. However, like all conventional drug therapies, there are side effects, and for some patients these can become an issue, with many sufferers unable to take the drugs for various reasons, e.g. pregnancy.

It should also be noted that in many cases, the drugs simply do not clear the infestation and the parasite maintains its grip despite all conventional attempts to remove it. Re-infestation is also an issue because doctors do not promote the need for partners and/or family members to be checked for infection, so the parasite just keeps circulating via individuals in the group.

Follow-up testing is not routinely offered after treatment either, so although the parasite may have been sufficiently weakened to ensure a respite from symptoms occurs, it will not be long before it recovers and re-infests the host once the treatment has finished.

It is generally these patients who end up in my consulting room.

The allopathic approach

Antibiotics are conventionally used to treat sufferers of giardiasis, and a doctor will, if appropriate for the patient, prescribe one of the drugs listed below. The prognosis is usually good; however, resistance to treatment and re-infection can occur.

Metronidazole (Flagyl)

Metronidazole is the antibiotic drug of choice for treating giardiasis (not suitable during pregnancy or breastfeeding). It works by entering and interfering with genetic material (DNA) in the cells of the parasite and prevents it from forming new DNA. This ultimately kills off the parasite and clears up the infection. The recommended adult dose is 400 mg three times daily for five days.

Some of the side effects associated with taking metronidazole can be the same or similar to the symptoms of giardiasis – such as, feeling sick, vomiting, stomach pain, hot flushes, a pounding heartbeat (palpitations) and headache.[2]

Tinidazole (Tindamax)

Tinidazole works in a similar way to metronidazole but has a longer duration of action. It should not be taken during the first trimester of pregnancy, and breast feeding should be avoided during and for three days after completing the treatment. The recommended adult dose is 2 grams once a day. Some of the very common side effects of this drug are loss of appetite, furred tongue, gastrointestinal disturbances, nausea, oral mucositis (mouth ulceration), taste disturbance and vomiting.

Both metronidazole and tinidazole are the treatment of choice for giardiasis and both produce similar results, but there was a 15.1% treatment failure in the UK in 2008, increasing in 2013 to 40.2%, with patients coming mainly from India and the Mediterranean in the study.[3] So, is Giardia becoming resistant to these antibiotics?

Quinacrine (Atabrine)

Quinacrine is an anti-protozoal drug originally used to treat and suppress malaria. It has also been used as an antibiotic to treat giardiasis. The exact mechanism of its antiparasitic action is unknown, but it appears to interfere with the parasite's metabolism and, like metronidazole and tinidazole, destroys its DNA and inhibits its renewal, destroying the Giardia's ability to survive.

Quinacrine is used for patients who are resistant to metronidazole as well as those who cannot take it – that is, women in the first three months of pregnancy, or those who are allergic to metronidazole or any of its ingredients. In chronic cases, where giardiasis is not responding to metronidazole alone, patients may be given a combination of quinacrine and metronidazole.[4]

The recommended adult dose of quinacrine to treat giardiasis is 100 mg every eight hours for five to seven days.

Side effects include gastrointestinal disturbances, dizziness, headache and yellow discolouration of skin, sclera (the white outer layer of the eyeball) and urine, due to it being a yellow dye which builds up concentration in the liver.

Many of the patients I see who are suffering from giardiasis could be classed as chronic sufferers, with years of failed attempts by various practitioners, to diagnose the problem, deal with it, and help restore their gut to normal working.

My experience is that while conventional medicines can be effective against giardiasis, from what my patients tell me, they are often poorly informed about the risks of re-infection and cross-infection, and how these may occur. For example, very rarely are patients told how prolific the Giardia parasite is and that all those living in close proximity to the patient need to be checked for infection, not just their partners. Most vets, when diagnosing an animal infected with Giardia, will recommend treating all the animals in the household because they know how quickly Giardia will find another host in close proximity. It is surprising to me this advice is not given by practitioners treating humans suffering from this condition.

The malaria link

During my 20 plus years of treating patients suffering from a Giardia infestation, I have tried many different combinations of herbs from all over the world, but the principal herb I now use to treat giardiasis is *Artemisia annua*. It is commonly known as 'sweet wormwood' and has proven, time and time again in my practice, to be extremely effective against Giardia.

Artemisia annua is native to China and interestingly, is the herb the Chinese have used for many years to treat malaria. In 2006, the World Health Organization (WHO), in collaboration with the Chinese government, published a document called *Monograph on Good Agricultural and Collection Practices (GACP) for Artemisia annua*,[5] which serves as a guide to other countries wishing to cultivate the plant for its medicinal value in treating malaria. The document also confirms the plant has been used in Chinese Herbal Medicine for over 2000 years to treat malaria.

Like giardiasis, malaria is caused by a parasitic infection, which is spread by the female Anopheles mosquitos. The plasmodium parasite (*Plasmodium falciparum*), that causes malaria, is single-celled and multiplies in the red blood cells of humans as well as in the mosquito intestine.

Malaria is a complex disorder and there are many strains, which all react differently to treatment. Artemisinin is a compound formulated from the *Artemisia annua* herb and the WHO recommends artemisinin-based combination therapies (ACTs) for the treatment of 'uncomplicated' malaria strains.[6] An ACT is made up of the drug artemisinin and a partner drug, and although there are obvious differences between giardiasis and malaria, a study carried out in 2016 noted that artemisinin and its derivaties were not only combating malaria, but were also successfully impacting various parasitic protozoa and this included *Giardia lamblia*.[7] The study concluded more work needed to be carried out before a clinical application could be made but this study lends weight to my own experience of successfully treating Giardia infestations with *Artemisia annua*, and this next story illustrates the point.

Sally's story

This is what Sally told me at our first consultation:

I came back from travelling in Kenya, Africa, in May 2007 and became very ill with vomiting, diarrhoea and water retention. These symptoms started approximately three weeks after my return from Africa. This trip lasted for five months and I was perfectly well during that time. It was after my return that I started to feel unwell.

I had been taking antimalarial tablets – Larium (mefloquine) –

which I had started two weeks before my departure to Kenya, and which I stopped taking two weeks after my return home. It was shortly after this that the bowel symptoms occurred.

I was diagnosed by my doctor three months later as having giardiasis and was given a four-day course of the antibiotic Metronidazole, and the severity of the symptoms stopped. However, since then my stomach/bowels have never been 'right'. I go through cycles of random vomiting or diarrhoea about every three months. I seem to feel bloated and have stomach pains on a daily basis that are quite intrusive in daily life and I can also be constipated for up to five days at a time. The doctor said it was probably irritable bowel syndrome (IBS) and so I took some over-the-counter pills, but they did not help. There is no one thing that seems to aggravate the condition. It seems to go in cycles of one week worse than another, but with no common factor causing it. The stools can have an offensive smell, sometimes with mucus.

When Sally came to see me, I diagnosed Giardia in her small intestine and gallbladder. I also detected she had developed a sensitivity to gluten.

I gave her a dietary protocol to follow for a few weeks, which included cutting out gluten from her diet, and prescribed my wormwood tincture to deal with the Giardia, together with herbs to support the gallbladder.

Sally returned the following week and all her symptoms had greatly improved. She continued with the treatment for another week and was eventually discharged from my care once the infection had cleared. I saw her a year later when she returned because she had been infected again with Giardia. Sally was a student teacher and working in schools can be a high-risk area for contracting this parasite.

Treating Giardia with herbs

When treating a case of giardiasis, chronic or acute, I usually find the sufferer has other debilitating issues which have manifested as a result of this infestation. Supporting and restoring a weakened digestive system, and all the dependent organs and processes which have been compromised, is also undertaken using the many herbal remedies I have formulated over the years for this very purpose. The success of the treatment also depends very much on the quality of the herbs used and the dosage taken.

Many herbs are bitter tasting, which is beneficial to health as it stimulates the digestive system, clearing sluggish waste and creating an environment which parasites do not like. However, sweet tasting foods are the everyday norm, and the bitterness of herbs may be difficult for children to take because they are unfamiliar with the taste. Also, if a person has liver problems then taking herbal tinctures, which contain alcohol, is contraindicated; alternative methods can be offered, such as herbal teas.

As mentioned earlier, *Artemisia annua* (sweet wormwood) is my treatment of choice for giardiasis. To eliminate the Giardia parasite, a fresh plant tincture is best, but a tincture made from dried herbs can work well provided they are of good quality and come from a reputable supplier. A tincture of wormwood is made by steeping the fresh herb in a solution of ethyl alcohol and water for approximately two to three weeks, stirring daily. Taken internally, it works best as a single tincture and not mixed with other herbs. My recommended dose is 10 ml of wormwood in 20 ml of water, taken three times a day, before meals, but this depends on the weight and size of the patient. Children and fragile individuals will need less.

Giardia can be more active at night, as the parasite feeds and breeds, so the last dose should be taken before going to bed.

Infusion of dried *Artemisia annua*

As I have said, occasionally, alcohol is a problem for some people, therefore a decoction of the dried herb is required. The adult dose is 10 grams per day and it is made in the following way.

Method

1. Soak 10 grams of dried *Artemisia annua* herb in 500 ml of water for one hour.
2. Bring to the boil and simmer gently for 20 minutes (do not allow to boil dry).
3. Strain the liquid, let it cool, and drink half in the morning and the remaining half in the evening.

Note: Wormwood and any accompanying herbs should be taken under the guidance of a qualified medical herbalist and the dosages should not be exceeded. They should not be taken with steroids or antibiotics. Please consult a doctor if taking any medication.

If I detect Giardia's presence in a patient's gallbladder, sinus or pancreas, I will also prescribe specific herbs for these areas to be taken in conjunction with the wormwood.

Herbal sprays

Some years ago, I developed a unique system of delivery for all the herbal treatments I use which allows me to offer my remedies to patients who may be unable to ingest the tinctures or herbal infusions for various reasons. Each of my remedies can be administered in a spray form, and enters the body via the etheric energetic field (see Chapter 12). This system is gentle, supportive, non-invasive and effective, perfect for treating children and adults alike.

I use this method for treating many of the patients I see, not just those suffering from giardiasis, and the results are the same, if not better than, when the herbs are ingested. A spray has the advantage of the remedy bypassing the digestive system with all its processes and chemicals, and gently helps the body to a balanced state of health.

Whether taking herbal tinctures, infusions or using the

sprays externally, signs of improvement vary from individual to individual; however, this treatment does not need to be taken over a long period, and I have observed complete recovery in a week in some cases.

I'd like to finish this chapter by sharing another story. This is from 'Ann' and shows just how disruptive to normal life Giardia can be if it is not diagnosed and eradicated quickly.

Ann's story

In August 2013, I travelled to India and on my return, I started having loose stools in the morning. This gradually got worse and eventually I lost my appetite; I could not even look at food. I started getting horrendous sulphur burps, and then the gurgling started. My stools were yellow liquid, incredibly bad smelling, almost chemical. They were oily, and they floated.

Even after two courses of metronidazole, my symptoms returned and lasted for two months. Although my appetite eventually came back, I was still running to the toilet up to 20 times a day, at times every 20 minutes. The symptoms were not improving on their own. The doctors assured me the parasite was gone and that I could be like this for up to a year whilst my body recovered. Three different GPs misdiagnosed me. However, I was not convinced, so I visited the drop-in clinic at the London Hospital for Tropical Diseases, where I tested positive for Giardia in a stool sample.

I was put on a course of antibiotics (tinidazole) and my symptoms stopped after only a few hours. I could eat and drink what I wanted with no signs of having ever been ill. I was over the moon. I fell pregnant soon after this and had a healthy happy pregnancy.

Then, two weeks after giving birth, my symptoms returned again – but this time they were worse. I was vomiting violently, producing sulphur burps and running to the toilet every half hour. I was unable to do anything. I managed to get another prescription for tinidazole and once again my symptoms vanished within hours. The doctors did not want to investigate *the reccurrence of Giardia despite my concerns about it returning again.*

I remained symptom free for a year and then in July 2015 the problem returned. However, this time it had changed. I was sick, yet did not lose my appetite. I had mild sulphur burps and bloating. I had loose pale stools followed by constipation. This was when I first consulted Susan over a Skype call and used her Giardia spray alongside a week-long course of herbs. My symptoms improved greatly, however, I was not sure if the parasite was totally gone as I had some bloating etc. I also developed unrelenting tinnitus in my ears as well as sinus issues.

For another year I appeared to be free of the parasite. I did have five episodes of vomiting which did not appear to be related to illness but rather to problems with my digestion. I started to think I had perhaps developed food intolerances. Then in July 2016, I started to have loose stools in the morning; I then lost my appetite and started to get sulphur burps and liquid yellow diarrhoea with the same smell and greasy floating consistency. I was also violently sick and my food was coming back up totally undigested although it had been in my stomach for over 12 hours. Without a doubt the parasite was back. I managed to secure another course of the antibiotics and my symptoms stopped. Unfortunately, this time it was different; the symptoms came back immediately after I stopped the treatment. The antibiotic was becoming ineffective.

After this episode I had periods of total loss of appetite, loose/liquid stools, constipation, pale stools, stomach cramps, extreme fatigue, depression, bloating and, immediately after eating, extreme gurgling and burping.

I went back to Susan and I discussed the possibility of being re-infected. As a teacher, I come into contact with hundreds of children a day. I can mark their work during my lunch break, therefore touching students' work while I am eating – the chance of re-infection is high.

I tested positive again for Giardia and I was given some more herbs – the treatment worked within a few days and I now keep one of the sprays in my medicine cabinet just in case!

Summary

The standard antiobiotic treatment for giardiasis can be successful, but sometimes the infection is not completely eradicated and re-infection occurs. It is important that retesting on completion of the treatment is done to ensure the parasite is no longer present. Herbs can also be very effective, but again, careful monitoring of the patient throughout the treatment goes a long way to achieving the desired result.

Taking medicines orally may not always be possible and the next chapter explains how herbal sprays can work just as well, and with no side effects.

Chapter 12

Healing through energy fields

I have always been interested in what is generally known as 'energy healing', and yet most people, if asked, would be hard pressed to explain what that actually is. I do not intend to immerse my readers in lengthy explanations regarding this subject, or discuss the amazing array of practitioners working in this field, but it is important to expand just a little on the scientific backdrop supporting the many energy healing modalities that exist today.

As western scientists and biologists have known for some time, the human body, with all its trillions of cells, atoms and protons, is simply a collection of coherent information and energy, vibrating at a particular rate and frequency which, when tapped into, can provide valuable information about its overall wellbeing.

Everything has a vibrational frequency which is measured in Hertz (Hz) and these electromagnetic frequencies have been researched for over a hundred years. Even the heartbeat of the planet has been detected, and is measured at 7.8 Hz. The physicist Winfried Otto Schumann predicted it mathematically in 1952 and it is known as the Schumann Cavity Resonance.[1]

Ampere's Law of Physics states that when currents flow through human tissue, energy fields are created in the surrounding space called 'bio-magnetic fields'. In 1903, Willem

Einthoven, a Dutch doctor and physiologist, invented the first practical electrocardiogram and, in 1924, he received a Nobel Prize for his discovery of its mechanism.[2]

Electrocardiograms are used by cardiologists and in clinics throughout the world, to check the electrical activity of the heart and to make clinical decisions on the information they provide. In 1929, the German scientist Hans Berger's research on the electrical fields of the brain, using electrodes on the skin surface to record electrical frequencies, led to the development and refinement of the technique known today as electroencephalography (EEG). Medical research now uses a magnetometer called a 'superconducting quantum interference device' (or 'SQID'), to study the human energy field, which provides more information than the aforementioned electrocardiograms and electroencephalograms.

We also know that for centuries many Eastern philosophies and cultures around the globe have named and talked about a 'light body' or 'aura' surrounding the human body and that this 'light body' is made up of various layers, all of which have a specific function in maintaining the health and wellbeing of the physical body. This 'aura' has even been photographed using a process called Kirlian photography which was discovered in 1939 by Semyon Kirlian, using a process which allowed him to capture the field surrounding living things.

We live in exciting times and, today, medicine and the conventional approach to healing are changing. Mainstream science is embracing new concepts in relation to the biological make-up of all life and in this shifting paradigm the concept of biofields is emerging which combines our understanding of the complex chemical biology of all living systems with the increasing evidence that an organising energy field is present and engaged in all aspects of healing and the healthy maintenance of all life.[3]

The concept of a holistic energy system, permeating all organisms living and inert, has been at the heart of eastern cultures for centuries and is known as *Qi (chi)*, or *prana*, in the various healing modalities practised.

My long-time interest in the energetic fields associated with the human body, and their relevance and importance to good health, led me to Dr Barbara Ann Brennan, an American physicist, author and teacher. Dr Brennan worked as a physicist for NASA and has devoted 35 years to the research and exploration of the human energy field. Her first book, *Hands of Light: A Guide to Healing Through the Human Energy Field*, is considered a classic in energy healing and explains in great detail the workings of the subtle energetic layers, or bodies as they are known, which make up the human aura. According to Dr Brennan, and others working in this field, each subtle energetic body impacts the functioning and wellbeing of all systems in the physical body, and by working with the unique frequencies of these energy bodies it is possible to impact the overall health of the physical body we all see and experience.

The main subtle bodies are:

1. The Etheric Body
2. The Emotional Body
3. The Mental Body
4. The Astral Level
5. The Etheric Template Body
6. The Celestial Body
7. The Causal Body or Ketheric Template.

The etheric body

The first of the subtle energetic bodies is called the 'etheric body' and is the one closest to the physical body. It is an energetic 'blueprint' of the physical body and Dr Brennan suggests this 'body' exists prior to cells developing. The 'etheric' body is the one I will focus on in this chapter since it is the one I interact with mostly when treating my patients – it is also the delivery system for the sprays I use in my practice to treat a number of complaints, including giardiasis.

It is possible for the experienced eye to see the etheric body; it looks like grey smoke or a heat haze whisping just a few centimeters upwards from the body. Its primary role is to deliver the life force energy to the physical body and it is the densest of all the energy bodies – its aura extends about 1 inch (2.5 cm) from the physical body.

The flow of energy to the physical body is affected by how we think and feel. Depression is a classic example of this phenomenon as we see the life force and vitality diminish in people we know who are dealing with this debilitating condition.

Another interesting fact I discovered about the etheric body, in my early work with energy, is that even if an organ or a limb is missing, or has been surgically removed, the energetic blueprint of that organ or limb will remain in the etheric field and can become a source of blocked energy, producing pain. We have all heard of people who have lost limbs suffering pain in the area where the limb used to be, and my experience shows that when an organ, such as the gallbladder, kidney or womb, is removed, the energy field of the missing body part is still present and can be re-energised and strengthened with my herbal remedies. Using my spray technique, and the appropriate herbs, I can treat the whole area affected so healing can take place. This encounter I had with a patient is a good illustration of that fact.

David's story

David came to me when he had lost two fingers in an accident at work. The surgeons had tried to re-attach the digits but this was unsuccessful. He was in a lot of pain where the fingers had been and he felt as though they were still there; this is known as 'phantom pain'.

The rest of his hand felt numb and he couldn't feel energy flowing through the damaged tissues around the injury. In

Chapter 12

Chinese Herbal Medicine theory, energy and blood flow together and blocked energy creates stagnation of blood, which in turn creates pain. The remedy I used included herbs for shock and trauma, blood moving and bones and joints.

The next day, David reported that the pain was greatly diminished and his hand felt more comfortable.

The *chakras*

Dr Brennan's work also details the existence and function of what she calls 'transformers'. These are spinning energy centres which are positioned in specific places along the body. Each of these energy vortices takes in the universal life force energy, and circulates it throughout all the subtle energy bodies, nourishing, healing, energising and maintaining health in a holistic fashion. In eastern philosophies these energy centres are known as *chakras* and for a strong, clear, balanced energy system, the *chakras* need to be in harmony to allow the life force energy (*Qi* or *prana*, as I've said) to flow unencumbered to all parts of the body.

The concept of *chakras* dates back to at least 2000 BC and is mentioned in the *Vedas*, which are ancient Hindu texts. These were written largely by the Aryans. The Aryans were said to have invaded India on chariots, and the original meaning of the word *chakra* as 'wheel' refers to their chariot wheels.

Traditional writings say there are some 88,000 *chakras* in the human body and each of these regulates, connects and affects the energetic flow in different areas of the physical body.

There are seven primary *chakras*, and they are located along a central vertical axis of our spine, and open out toward the front of the body. Like Dr Brennan's 'transformers', these circular energy centres are in constant motion, spinning, attracting, receiving or radiating energy, and each one has a specific vibration and sphere of influence within the body. They also have specific physical, psychological, emotional, spiritual and energetic characteristics. The amount of energy the *chakras* draw in is regulated and balanced by the needs of the body to maintain vitality, health and general wellbeing in the individual areas of influence. Western research has shown that imbalances in the 'transformers', or *chakras*, are an indication of dis-ease in the specific area governed by a weak or imbalanced *chakra*.[4]

Here are the seven primary *chakras*, where they are located in the body and their unique sphere of influence.

The base chakra is situated in the pelvic plexus at the base of the spine and relates to the bladder, colon, adrenal glands, spine and lower back.

The sacral chakra is situated at the sacrum and relates to the hips, sacrum, lower back, kidneys, prostate and reproductive organs, and affects menstruation and semen production.

The solar plexus chakra is situated just below the navel and relates to the middle back, stomach, intestines, pancreas, liver and gallbladder.

The heart chakra is situated just in front of the heart and relates to the thymus gland, lymph glands, heart and circulatory system, upper back, shoulders and arms.

The throat chakra is situated at the base of the throat and relates to the thyroid gland, parathyroid, larynx, throat, tongue, mouth and teeth.

The third-eye chakra is situated between the eyebrows and relates to the sinus, ears and eyes.

The crown chakra is situated just above the head and relates to the brain, cerebral cortex, pituitary gland, pineal gland, nervous system and skin.

As discussed, the spin of each *chakra* in the human body is unique, and is dependent on the physical, emotional and spiritual environment surrounding them being in harmony. It is believed, if we lead a simple, peaceful life with daily exercise, meditation and prayer, we will keep the *chakras* rotating at their correct velocity and prevent dis-ease from entering our body. Honestly speaking, how many of us can say, in the turbulent times of modern life, this is how we live? Not many, and we, as humans, have had to adapt to life in the 21st century with all its technology, stress, crazy diets and dependence on pharmaceuticals to keep us going.

I accept it is not always possible to address these issues, but the key is to try and maintain a balance in life and take control of whatever we can. Our food, our stress, our emotional health and our happiness all play a major part in maintaining this balance and we need to be mindful of their importance if we want to live a long and healthy life.

When things get out of balance 'dis-ease' can set in, and since we know everything has a measurable vibrational frequency, including the Giardia parasite, it is not too big a leap to see that altering the vibrational frequency at the affected part of the body could eliminate the invader and restore the balance of energy so our body can heal itself. Remember, if the environment does not suit the pathogen then it will not survive and flourish. However, these invaders are great at adapting their environment to suit their needs, so we have to adopt a healthy and low-stress lifestyle and listen to what our bodies are telling us.

My sprays

I have briefly mentioned my sprays in previous chapters and as they are an integral part of my clinical practice, a deeper explanation of what they are and how they work is offered here for clarity.

Early on in my clinical work, I often encountered patients who were unable to ingest my herbal remedies and tinctures for a variety of reasons so I needed to develop a protocol of delivery which could by-pass the digestive system. I began my research by looking at the seven primary *chakras* as a way of accessing the energetic fields surrounding the physical body and its organs. I wanted to see if it was possible to draw the therapeutic essences of my herbal formulas into the body, for absorption at a cellular level, and see what, if any, impact this would have on treating Giardia. I worked with the knowledge that the *chakras* are spiralling vortices, like tornados, and by spraying into the centre of the *chakra*, the herbal essences would be drawn down to the cellular level where they would weaken the Giardia and its cysts by changing the vibration and therefore the environment. This would ensure the parasite could no longer thrive and flourish and, would cause it quickly to perish. I have applied this technique of treatment over a number of years, with many of my patients, and have observed its success consistently. It is clear to me my sprays work through the energetic bodies to deliver treatment, and my tinctures and teas work directly with the physical body.

How to use the sprays

All of my sprays are formulated to work in the same way as the Giardia spray, and, depending on the physical problem and the treatment plan I recommend, the following instructions apply:

- The herbal spray must be shaken near the patient for five seconds to synchronise the vibrational levels of the herbs to the individual and create resonance.
- The spray should be delivered in five short bursts, in the appropriate *chakra*, from approximately 30 cm.
- Young children and the very elderly may need less.
- If spraying through clothes, it is advisable to spray through a tissue so staining from the herbs is avoided.
- These sprays can also be applied directly onto the skin, but any concerns regarding contact with the skin can be avoided by using a tissue.

The protocol I have developed for treating Giardia, and most of the other complaints my patients present with, is unique, effective and does not interfere with other medication being taken. It also does not offend children's taste buds, is simple and quick to administer, and can be carried around in hand luggage, just in case we should pick up Giardia on our travels.

It is important to remember the sprays are strictly for external use only and should be kept out of the reach of children and stored away from direct sunlight.

Conclusion

I hope you have found this information useful, helpful and enlightening. It is my view we have to find new ways of facing the health challenges of 21st-century life on this planet – our health professionals and state services are becoming overwhelmed with people suffering from chronic conditions for which there seem to be no remedies. New doctors are aware 70% of the people they will encounter in their surgeries will be suffering from these chronic complaints, and they will be unable to help them – a disappointing prospect for a newly qualified medic.

I believe a crisis is an evolutionary driver and unless we find new, innovative and holistic ways of dealing with our health challenges, which encompass the beauty and magnificence of all our natural resources, we will have a greatly curtailed future as a species on this glorious planet.

Appendices

Appendix I

Herbs

Throughout the evolution of our planet, plants have been growing which contain everything required to balance and maintain our health – it is just a matter of knowing which ones to use, and how to prepare them. Knowledge of herbs and their medicinal properties has been passed down from generation to generation, in cultures all around the world, while other animals have a natural instinct to seek out particular plants in order to self-medicate. Herbal products have become a popular sight in many of our local shops and supermarkets, and yet few of us understand the ancient wisdom behind them, wisdom which our forebears grew up with.

Throughout this book I have made reference to health issues which can accompany an infestation of Giardia, and which I am also able to treat with my herbal formulations. The most common of these issues affect the gallbladder, the pancreas, the kidneys and the sinuses. The tinctures and teas I formulate involve the use of many herbs, some of which are well known, others not so much. For those readers interested in knowing more about these herbs, I have included information here about some of those I use when dealing with Giardia.

In the list that follows I have used the terminology that is specific to herbal medicines ('carminative', etc). Rather than explain these on all occasions, please turn to the Glossary for the meaning – or just click there and back if you're reading the ebook.

It is important to note, medicinal herbs, like pharmaceutical drugs, may have side effects if taken in an unregulated and unsupervised manner, and should only be administered by a qualified herbalist or other appropriately trained health professional.

Glossary of herbs

ANISEED

> **Botanical name:** *Pimpinella anisum*
> **Plant family:** Umbelliferae
> **Part used:** Dried fruit
> **Constituents:** Volatile oils, fatty acids
> **Actions:** Expectorant, antispasmodic, carminative, parasiticide, aromatic
> **Medicinal use:** The volatile oil is excellent for easing griping pains and flatulence.

BARBERRY

> **Botanical name:** *Berberis vulgaris*
> **Plant family:** Berberidaceae
> **Parts used:** Bark of root, fresh or dried, stem bark, berries
> **Constituents:** Alkaloids (berberine), tannins
> **Actions:** Cholagogue, astringent and bitter tonic, anti-protozoal, anti-pyretic
> **Medicinal use:** Barberry acts on the gallbladder to improve bile flow and is used to reduce gallbladder pain and jaundice.

BOLDO

> **Botanical name:** *Peumus boldo*
> **Plant family:** Monimiaceae

Part used: Leaves
Constituents: Volatile oil, alkaloid, resins, tannins
Actions: Anthelmintic, antioxidant, chologogue, choleretic, diuretic, hepato-protective
Medicinal use: Treatment for gallstones and gallbladder inflammation (cholecystitis, hepatitis and worm infestations).

CAYENNE, CHILLI

Botanical name: *Capsicum minimum*
Plant family: Solanaceae
Part used: Fruit
Constituents: Alkaloid, carotenoids, vitamin C
Actions: Stimulant, tonic, carminative, antiseptic, analgesic, antispasmodic
Medicinal use: The fruits are used to increase sweating and to encourage the release of toxins by increasing blood flow to the skin.

CENTAURY

Botanical name: *Erythraea centarium*
Plant family: Gentianaceae
Part used: Herb
Constituents: Glycosidal bitter principles, volatile oil, resin
Actions: Bitter, aromatic, mild nervine, gastric stimulant
Medicinal use: For treatment of sluggish digestive system, loss of appetite and dyspepsia.

CHAMOMILE, GERMAN

Botanical name: *Matricaria recutita*
Plant family: Compositae
Parts used: The flowers
Constituents: Volatile oils which include chamazulene,

courmarin, flavone glycosides

Actions: Anti-spasmodic, carminative, anti-inflammatory, analgesic, antiseptic, vulnerary

Medicinal use: Gentle sedative action which is safe for children and is useful for treating anxiety and insomnia. Also used to treat stomach ulcers and as a gargle for quinsy and sore, inflamed gums and throat.

CHAPARREL, CREOSOTE BUSH

Botanical name: *Larrea tridentate*
Plant family: Zygophylloceae
Part used: Aerial parts
Constituents: Lignans, flavonoid glycosides, protein
Actions: Antiviral, antibacterial, antifungal, anti-inflammatory, antioxidant, antibiotic
Medicinal use: Aids the treatment of colds, sinusitis and pain associated with arthritis.

CINNAMON

Botanical name: *Cinnamomum zeylanicum*
Plant family: Lauraceae
Part used: Dried inner bark
Constituents: Volatile oils, tannins, terpenes
Actions: Spasmolytic, carminative, anti-diarrhoeal, antimicrobial
Medicinal use: Used in the treatment of bronchitis, and to help lower blood sugar levels.

CLOVE

Botanical name: *Syzigium aromaticum*
Plant family: Myrtaceae
Parts used: Dried flowers and oil
Constituents: Up to 20% volatile oil

Actions: Antiseptic, antispasmodic
Indications: Carminative, astringent, aromatic, stimulant
Medicinal use: Cloves have been used in Southeast Asia for thousands of years as a panacea for all ailments. In a study it was shown that cloves improve glucose, cholesterol and triglycerides in people with type 2 diabetes mellitus.[1] It can be used as a mild anaesthetic for aching teeth.

COUCHGRASS

Botanical name: *Agropyron repens*
Plant family: Graminaceae
Part used: The rhizome
Constituents: Mucilage, potassium, silicic acid, inositol, glycoside
Actions: Diuretic, demulcent, antimicrobial
Medicinal use: For treatment of cystitis, prostatitis, kidney stones and gravel, and its demulcent properties reduce inflammation.

ECHINACEA

Common name: *Echinacea angustofolia*
Plant family: Compositae
Part used: Cone flower
Constituents: Volatile oil, glycoside, phenols
Actions: Antimicrobial, alterative
Medicinal use: Echinacea is effective in both bacterial and viral attacks and is especially useful for sinus problems

When I went to China to study herbal medicine in Beijing, half of our group came down with a bad cough. I had decided to take Echinacea as a preventative and even though my room-mate had the Beijing cough I stayed clear from the infection. One other person in the group also took Echinacea and, like me, she did not get infected.

ELDER

Botanical name: *Sambucus nigra*
Plant family: Capriofoliaceae
Part used: Bark, flowers, berries, leaves
Constituents: Flavonoids, tannins, essential oil, vitamin C in the berries
Actions: Bark – Purgative, emetic, diuretic; Leaves – Externally, emollient and vulnerary; Flowers – Diaphoretic, anti-catarrhal; Berries – Diaphoretic, diuretic, laxative
Medicinal use: Elder flowers are excellent in the treatment of colds and influenza and useful for upper respiratory catarrh.

FRINGE TREE

Botanical name: *Chionanthes virginicus*
Plant family: Oleaceae
Part used: Bark of roots and stem
Constituents: Saponin, glycoside
Actions: Alterative, cholagogue, bitter tonic, hepatic, laxative
Medicinal use: This bitter tonic is used to treat gallbladder and liver conditions.

GENTIAN

Botanical name: *Gentiana lutea*
Plant family: gentianaceae
Part used: The dried rhizome and root
Constituents: Bitter principles, pectin, tannin, mucilage, sugar
Actions: Bitter, gastric stimulant, sialogogue, cholagogue
Medicinal use: This is an excellent bitter which stimulates the appetite and is useful for sluggish digestion, dyspepsia and flatulence.

GINGER

Botanical name: *Zingiber officinalis*
Plant family: Zingiberaceae
Part used: The rootstock
Constituents: Volatile oils, starch, mucilage, resin
Actions: Stimulant, carminative, rubefacient, diaphoretic
Medicinal use: Ginger promotes digestion, dispels flatulence and colic, and suppresses vomiting.

GLOBE ARTICHOKE

Botanical name: *Cynara scolymus*
Plant family: Compositae
Part used: Leaves
Constituents: Flavonoids
Actions: Choleretic, diuretic
Medicinal use: Used in the prevention and treatment of gallstones and aids digestion.

GOAT'S RUE

Botanical name: *Galega officinalis*
Plant family: Leguminosae
Parts used: Aerial parts
Constituents: Alkaloids, saponins, flavones, glycosides, bitters, tannins
Actions: Anti-diabetic
Medicinal use: It has the ability to reduce blood sugar levels and can be helpful in the early stages of late onset diabetes.

GRAVEL ROOT

Common name: *Eupatorium purpureum*
Plant family: Compositae
Part used: Rhizome and root
Constituents: Volatile oil, resin, flavonoids

Actions: Diuretic, anti-lithic, anti-rheumatic
Medicinal use: Gravel root is used in the treatment of
kidney stones or gravel (small stones), cystitis and urethritis.

HYDRANGEA

Botanical name: *Hydrangea aborescens*
Plant family: Saxifragaceae
Part used: Dried root and rhizome
Constituents: Glycosides, saponins, resins
Actions: Diuretic, anti-lithic
Medicinal use: It is used in the treatment for enlarged
prostate, urinary stones or gravel (small stones) and cystitis.

LAVENDER

Botanical name: *Lavendeula officinalis*
Plant family: Labiate
Part used: Flowers
Constituents: Volatile oils
Actions: Carminative, anti-spasmodic, antidepressant,
rubefacient, antibacterial, antiseptic
Medicinal use: Lavender is very calming and soothing and
useful for treating headaches. The oil can help in the healing
of burns.

LEPTANDRA

Botanical name: *Leptandra virginicus*
Plant family: Scrophulariaceae
Part used: Dried rhizome, roots
Constituents: The roots contain volatile oil, tannic acid, gum
and resin
Actions: Cathartic, emetic
Medicinal use: Leptandra gently stimulates the liver and
promotes the secretion of bile.

MARIGOLD

Botanical name: *Calendula officinalis*
Plant family: Compositae
Part used: Yellow petal (florets)
Constituents: Saponins, carotenoids, essential oil, flavonoids
Actions: Anti-inflammatory, astringent, vulnerary, anti-fungal, cholagogue, emmenagogue
Medicinal use: Reduces inflammation of mucous membranes and aids healing.

MYRRH

Botanical name: *Commiphora molmol*
Plant family: Burseraceae
Parts used: Gum, resin
Constituents: Essential oil, up to 40% resin, gums
Actions: Antimicrobial, astringent, carminative,anti-catarrhal, expectorant
Medicinal use: Myrrh is very beneficial for treating mouth ulcers, gingivitis and pyorrhea,(infection of the ligaments and bones that support the teeth), and also for respiratory complaints, sinusitis and pharyngitis.

NEEM TREE

Botanical name: *Azadirachta indica*
Plant family: Meliaceae
Parts used: Seeds, leaves, flowers, stem and stem bark
Constituents: Terpenes, flavonoids, flavone glycoside
Actions: Antidiabetic, antifungal, antiviral, antibacterial
Medicinal use: The neem tree has been used in Ayurvedic medicine to treat a wide variety of ailments, including worms in the gut. It has also been used as an insect repellent, the treatment of head lice and in India the end of a neem stick is chewed and used as a toothbrush. Neem is also used in toothpastes.

NETTLE

Botanical name: *Urtica dioica*
Plant family: Urticacea
Parts used: Aerial parts
Constituents: Histamine, formic acid, chlorophyll, iron, vitamin C
Actions: Astringent, diuretic, tonic
Medicinal use: The seeds are used to help support the kidneys. The astringent action helps stop bleeding and it is a good general tonic.

OREGON GRAPE

Botanical name: *Berberis aquifolium*
Plant family: Berberideaceae
Part used: Root
Constituents: Alkaloids
Medicinal use: Oregon grape is very useful in helping to clear catarrah from the head and sinus regions; it is also used for treating gastritis.

PELLITORY OF THE WALL

Botanical name: *Parietaria officinalis*
Plant family: Urticaceae
Parts used: Aerial parts
Constituents: Bitter principle, tannins
Actions: Diuretic, demulcent
Medicinal use: Pellitory is useful for treating cystitis and pyelitis (inflammation of the lining of the renal pelvis of the kidney), as well as kidney stones and gravel.

PEPPERMINT

Botanical name: *Mentha piperita*
Plant family: Labiate

Parts used: Aerial parts
Constituents: Volatile oil; tannins, bitter principle
Actions: Carminative, anti-spasmodic, aromatic, diaphoretic, anti-emetic, nervine, antiseptic, analgesic
Medicinal use: Peppermint is useful in the treatment of fevers, and especially colds and influenza when mixed with elderberry and yarrow. It is also used for intestinal colic and flatulent dyspepsia.

PERIPLOCA OF THE WOOD (also called Gurmar)

Botanical name: *Gymnema sylvestre*
Plant family: Asclepiadaceae
Parts used: Leaves, roots
Constituents: Saponins, triterpenes, glycosides
Actions: Anti-hyperglycaemic , antiviral, antioxidant, cardiotonic, diuretic, laxative,
Medicinal use: In India this herb has been used in the treatment of diabetes mellitus and the name *gurmar* means 'sugar destroying' because if the leaves are chewed the taste of sugar and sweet substances disappears.

RED CLOVER

Botanical name: *Trifolium pretense*
Plant family: Papilionaceae
Parts used: Flowerheads
Constituents: Glycosides, flavonoids, coumarins, resins, minerals, vitamins
Actions: Alterative, expectorant, antispasmodic
Medicinal use: This is a blood cleanser and is used to treat skin conditions and breast cancer. Giardia need to attach to the mucosa (lining) of the small intestine to feed and red clover has been shown to inhibit attachment and movement of Giardia in 1.5 hours.[2]

STONE ROOT

Botanical name: *Colllinsonia canadensis*
Plant family: Labiate
Part used: Root and rhizome
Constituents: Saponins, tannin, resin, alkaloid
Actions: Anti-lithic, diuretic diaphoretic
Medicinal use: Stone root is used to treat stones in the urinary tract and gallbladder.

SWEET WORMWOOD

Botanical name: *Artemisia annua*
Plant family: Asteraceae
Parts used: Aerial parts, mainly the upper third of the plant which is highest in artemisinin
Consituents: Essential oils, artemisinin, flavonoids
Actions: Anti-protozoal, antibacterial and antioxidant
Medicinal use: This herb has been used for centuries for the treatment of malaria. Historically wormwood has been used as a parasitic worm killer.

THUJA

Botanical name: *Thuja occidentalis*
Plant family: Cupressaceae
Part used: Young twigs
Constituents: Volatile oil including thujone, flavonoids, glycoside, , mucilage, tannins
Actions: Expectorant, stimulant to smooth muscles, diuretic, astringent, alterative
Medicinal use: Used to treat bronchial catarrh due to its stimulating volatile oil.

THYMUS

Botanical name: *Thymus vulgaris*
Plant family: Labiatea
Parts used: Leaves and flowering tops
Constituents: Volatile oil, bitter principles, tannins, flavonoids, triterpenoids
Actions: Carminative, antimicrobial, antispasmodic, expectorant, astringent, anthelmintic
Medicinal use: It may be used to treat whooping cough, bronchitis and asthma and as a gargle for laryngitis and tonsillitis. In coughs it helps expectoration and reduces spasm.

WAHOO

Botanical name: *Eunonymous atropapeurins*
Plant family: Celastraceae
Parts used: Bark principally, but also the roots and berries
Constituents: Euonymol, euonysterol, atropurpurol, dulcitol, fatty acids
Actions: Anthelmintic, appetite stimulant, cholagogue, depurative, laxative
Medicinal use: Wahoo stimulates the gallbladder and liver and has a laxative effect. It is also used to treat worm infestations and skin disorders.

YARROW

Botanical name: *Achillea millefolium*
Plant family: Compositae
Part used: Aerial parts
Constituents: Volatile oil, flavonoids, tannins, bitter alkaloid
Actions: Diaphoretic, hypotensive, astringent, diuretic, antiseptic
Medicinal use: Yarrow is excellent for treating fevers, helping the body to sweat.

Appendix II

Glossary of terms

Aerial	part of the plant above ground
Alterative	cleansing removal of waste products
Analgesic	pain reliever
Anthelmintic	acts against parasitic worms
Antibacterial	destroys or suppresses bacteria
Antifungal	destroys fungus
Anti-hyperglycaemic	balances blood sugar
Anti-inflammatory	reduces inflammation or swelling
Anti-lithic	helps in the prevention of stones in the urinary tract and the elimination of stones already formed
Antioxidant	prevents cell damage
Anti-pyretic	brings temperature down
Antispasmodic	relieves muscle spasm
Antiviral	protects against viral attacks
Aromatic	having a pleasant smell
Astringent	contracts blood vessels and mucous membranes

Carminative	relieves flatulence and gastric discomfort
Cathartic	drastic purgative
Cholagogue	stimulates bile flow from the gallbladder and bile ducts
Choleretic	increases bile flow
Demulcent	soothes damaged or inflamed mucous membranes
Depurative	has purifying and detoxifying effects
Diaphoretic	encourages sweating
Emetic	induces vomiting
Emmenagogue	stimulates or increases menstrual flow
Expectorant	promotes the secretion of sputum
Hepatic	affects the liver
Hepato-protective	prevents damage to the liver
Mild nervine	mildly affects the nervous system either stimulating, relaxing or sedating
Parasiticide	destroys parasites
Rhizome	underground plant stem producing the roots and shoots of the new plant
Rubefacient	stimulates blood flow to the skin causing redness
Sialogogue	promotes secretion of saliva
Spasmolytic	relieves smooth muscle spasm
Vulnerary	heals wounds

Appendix III

Living without gluten

Many of my patients develop a sensitivity to gluten with the onset of giardiasis and need to omit it from their diet. I have, therefore, set out some guidelines for those considering going gluten-free for any period of time.

It is important to get to know the foods that are naturally gluten-free and they are:

- all meat, fish, fruit, vegetables and pulses – these can be eaten as long as they are not prepared with additives or seasonings that contain gluten.
- gluten-free breads, pastas and pastry options – there are plenty in most supermarkets these days, or for those who wish to make their own, there are many recipes with flours made from potato, rice, soy, amaranth, quinoa, buckwheat or beans, all of which are gluten free.

Food labels should be read carefully for ingredients that contain gluten.

The European Union Regulation No 828/2014[1] sets out the legal framework for the labelling of gluten-free and very low gluten food products. These regulations are quite specific as to what manufacturers and caterers need to be aware of as they apply to both packaged foods and those foods sold in catering establishments.

Eating out can be challenging, but many places now have a gluten-free menu if asked. Another option is to ask a waiter to find out from the chef how dishes are prepared to be sure they are gluten-free.

When invited to a friend's house, it is a good idea to let them know ahead of the event that gluten is an issue – much as vegetarians and vegans manage this problem.

Gluten-free grains

Rice

For those suffering from digestive problems, rice is an excellent and easily digestible food to include in the diet, and a staple food for at least half of the world's population – mostly in India, China, Japan and Southeast Asia.

Steamed coconut rice

This is one of my favourite ways of cooking and eating rice. I use:

one cup of long grain rice

one cup of freshly grated coconut

one cup of water

two tablespoons of coconut oil

¾ cup of coconut milk

(I make my own coconut milk using one cup of grated coconut blended with two cups of water until it is creamy)

Method

Brown the grated coconut in the coconut oil

Then add the dry rice and mix well

Add the coconut milk and water and bring to the boil

Stir it once, then cover and leave to simmer for 15 minutes

Remove it from the heat and leave covered for another five minutes

Fluff and serve.

Corn

Corn is also a useful food, although some coeliac patients cannot tolerate it. For those who can, it is a good replacement for wheat as a source of carbohydrates.[2]

Home-made popcorn

Popcorn is easy and quick to make, and is an excellent gluten-free snack. Make it fresh if possible, do not buy pre-popped. I use:

$1/3$ cup of corn kernels

3 tablespoons of coconut oil

1 pinch of salt or a knob of butter for extra flavour (optional).

Method

Melt the coconut oil in a heavy-based saucepan, over a medium heat

Test the temperature by throwing a few kernels in the pan; once these test kernels pop, throw in the others, cover with a tight lid, and remove from the heat

Wait 30 seconds and then return the pan to the heat and the popcorn should start popping

Shake the pan, and, when the popping slows down, remove it from the heat.

(Feel free to add more salt and/or butter to taste, shaking the pan so all the popcorn gets evenly covered.)

Buckwheat

Buckwheat is another alternative to rice. It can also be made into porridge and, contrary to popular belief, is not actually a grain but a fruit seed related to rhubarb and sorrel.

If eating grains is a problem, this is a good substitute, and highly nutritious. Buckwheat flour can be used for noodles or pancakes, or just to cook and have as a side dish.

Cooking buckwheat

Cover a cup of buckwheat with water, and soak it overnight. In the morning, rinse it thoroughly in a sieve before cooking in ½ cup of boiling water for three to five minutes, until it is soft.

Buckwheat is also nice left to cool and then made into a salad with chopped nuts, onions, peppers, and grated carrots, then seasoned with salt and lemon juice (optional).

Quinoa

Quinoa is a species of the goosefoot genus that is much more than a grain – it is actually a highly nutritious and very versatile combination of protein and gluten-free carbohydrate, great for stabilising blood sugar levels. Although it has relatively recently attained superfood status in the UK, it has been consumed for thousands of years in South America, and was an important crop for the Inca Empire who referred to it as the 'mother of all grains' and believed it to be sacred.

Cooking quinoa

Rinse one cup of quinoa under cold water and add to one and a half cups of water. Bring to the boil and cover, simmering gently until all the water has evaporated, approximately 15 minutes.

Millet

Millet is more than just a bird seed. I like to use it as a fluffy rice-like side dish. It is very high in B-vitamins, as well as calcium, iron, potassium, zinc and magnesium. However, a word of caution – millet should be eaten in moderation as it contains goitrogens, which can suppress thyroid activity.

It is delicious cooked as follows.

Cooking millet

One part millet to two parts water or broth

One pinch of salt (optional)

Knob of butter to stop the grains from sticking together (optional)

Method

Begin by toasting the seeds in a dry saucepan until they are golden brown

Then add in the liquid and salt and give it a stir

Bring to the boil and then add the butter

Simmer for about 15 minutes with the lid on

When removed from the heat, let the pan stand for about 10 minutes (like most grains, it needs a little time off the heat to fully absorb its cooking liquid)

When the lid is finally removed, fluff the millet with a fork, check the seasoning, and serve.

(For a millet porridge, increase the liquid to three parts.)

Couscous

Couscous is a popular alternative to rice and is available to buy as a millet-, barley- or sorghum-based couscous, as a gluten-free alternative to the usual semolina version (which is made from the hard part of the wheat grain).

Cooking couscous

Cook couscous in the same volume of boiling water – that is, one cup of couscous to one cup of boiling water. Add salt to taste, stir, and place in a pan for 10 minutes with the lid on until all the water has been absorbed and it is soft. Fluff with a fork and serve.

Sorghum

Sorghum is another ancient cereal grain and is a very important crop today due to its ability to withstand drought conditions. It is rich in phosphorus, magnesium, niacin, vitamin B6, iron and protein, and is a very useful whole grain to consider when looking for a natural gluten-free food as a substitute for wheat. It is also available to buy as flour.

Cooking sorghum

Cook one part sorghum grain in three parts of water, with 1 tablespoon of olive oil and a pinch of salt (optional). Bring it to the boil and then simmer until the grain is soft and chewy. This takes about an hour. If it's still too hard, add one more part of water and continue cooking.

Teff

This tiny poppy-seed-sized grain with its mild, nutty flavour, is high in protein and has the added advantage of containing calcium, magnesium and zinc, and can be ground into a flour for baking.

Cooking teff

Bring one cup of teff to the boil in three cups of water or stock, then simmer for 20 minutes.

Chia

Chia seeds, once used as currency by the Aztecs and Mayans because their high level of nutrients was so valuable, are another healthy gluten-free option, and can be eaten raw. Sprinkled onto any type of foods, they are quick, easy and nutritious.

Cooking chia

Chia seeds need no cooking but can be used raw to make a simple pudding. Just mix with coconut milk and berries, and chill overnight (use a container with a lid). The chia turns to gel as it swells and nuts and fresh fruit can also be added.

Conclusion

So whether you have giardiasis and cannot tolerate gluten, have been diagnosed with coeliac disease, or simply feel better on a gluten-free diet, this information is to help you live without gluten in your diet.

Please be aware that a number of different grains may be harvested, sorted and even packed in the same facilities. Often wheat flour may be in the atmosphere, or traces of it may be in the containers in which seeds such as chia are stored or transported, and, if suffering from coeliac disease or a severe gluten intolerance due to Giardia, even these small traces can trigger digestive problems.

Appendix IV

Maintaining a healthy gut microbiome

Giardia can play havoc with our digestion and even the healthiest of diets will be without value if the body cannot properly digest and assimilate its nutrients.

As discussed in Chapter 6, keeping our gut microbiome healthy is vital if we want to stay well, and eating a varied and balanced diet is one way we can do this. Common sense tells us that fresh fruit and vegetables are key to good health as they are high in fibre and will also provide many of the essential vitamins, minerals and nutrients required. Healthy fats and protein are also important, but carbohydrates should be included based on a person's energy requirements. Decreasing the intake of refined foods, sugar and alcohol, all of which have been shown to decrease resistance to infection, will have a dramatic and positive impact on our overall health, and will also help the body maintain a healthy gut microbiome.

Introduce fermented foods into your diet

Another way we can support our gut microbiome is to start consuming fermented foods. These are really good for the beneficial microbes in our gut; they contain 'probiotics', which are live beneficial bacteria that are naturally created during the fermentation process. Such foods include kefir, sauerkraut and 'live' natural yoghurt.

Kefir – a complex probiotic

Kefir is a fermented milk drink traditionally made from cows' or goats' milk and resembles yoghurt in appearance. It has large numbers of unique bacteria and yeast which distinguishes it from other probiotics.

Some of the benefits of kefir include:

- stimulates the immune system
- has anti-tumour properties
- contains bacteria that aid lactose (milk-sugar) digestion
- has antimicrobial properties
- regulates cholesterol, blood pressure and blood sugar
- has an anti-ageing effect due to its high quantities of antioxidants.

These benefits can be enjoyed from shop-bought kefir, but to really get the most benefit it is recommended you make your own. To do this you will need to obtain some kefir grains, which can be purchased as a Kefir starter kit. Here is a simple recipe.

Making your own kefir

You will need:

Plastic strainer (NOT metal)

1 glass jar (medium size)

A glass bowl

A plastic or wooden spatula (do not use metal)

Cheesecloth or paper towel

Rubber band

Kefir grains (living cultures), or a kefir starter kit

Milk (preferably raw, organic whole milk, but any milk will work)

Storage jar (kilner)

Method

Put 2-3 tablespoons of kefir grains to 2-3 cups of milk in the glass jar, leaving a space for the kefir to expand – for those who wish to remain on a dairy-free diet the milk can be substituted by coconut milk, apple juice or any other suitable medium.

Cover with the cheesecloth, and secure with the rubber band.

Store at room temperature for two days. During this time, it will thicken and separate; it should also smell sour. These are all signs it is ready.

Using the glass bowl and strainer, strain the liquid, stirring it to encourage it to separate.

When this has been done, there will be grains left in the strainer – put these leftover grains back into the jar and cover them with milk, for the next batch to start again.

Pour the newly made kefir into a storage jar with a lid, and keep it in the fridge.

Sauerkraut

Sauerkraut is another fermented food which contains beneficial probiotics. It is essentially fermented cabbage and also contains enzymes which help the body break down food which in turn helps us to absorb more nutrients. This recipe was given to me by a friend.

Receipe for sauerkraut

You will need:

2 cups shredded green cabbage

2 cups shredded red cabbage

1 tsp dried mustard

1 tsp caraway seeds or mustard seeds

1 tsp salt

1 garlic clove minced

1 tbs fresh lemon juice

1 cup filtered water

Method

In a glass bowl, combine the red and green cabbage, mustard seeds and salt.

In a separate small bowl, combine the garlic, lemon juice and filtered water.

Pour the mixture over the cabbage.

Cover the bowl, using clingfilm, and set aside at room temperature, for at least three days, shaking the bowl occasionally.

After this time, the sauerkraut is ready to transfer and store in jars in the fridge, for up to a year.

Immune-system boosting vitamins and minerals

Our immune system also needs an abundance of vitamins and minerals to keep it healthy. Here are some of the most important ones together with the foods in which the highest amounts are available:

- **Vitamin A** is important for improved vision, bone development, and as an immune stimulant – the main sources are found in carotenoid-rich carrots, spinach, sweet potatoes, red peppers, pumpkin, squash and apricots.
- **Vitamin C** is a good antioxidant and can be found in citrus fruit, red peppers, strawberries, tomatoes and

green vegetables such as broccoli and Brussels sprouts.

- **Vitamin E** dissolves blood clots, protects veins, and keeps the blood cells healthy – it can be found in nuts and seeds such as almonds, peanuts, pine nuts, hazelnuts, brazil nuts and sunflower seeds. If nuts are a problem, spinach, broccoli, olives, avocado and egg yolk are good sources.
- **Folate/folic acid (vitamin B9)** is important for brain function and plays an important part in mental and emotional health – it can be found in beans, peas, spinach, avocado and asparagus.
- **Iron** – has an important role in blood production. 'Haeme iron' is more easily absorbed from chicken, turkey and seafood. Beans, broccoli, kale, prunes and raisins are further good sources of iron.
- **Selenium** protects against oxidative stress and helps defend against heart disease and cancer – it is found in high quantities in Brazil nuts and the recommended daily allowance is obtained from just two of these nuts. Also, poultry and seafood contain selenium.
- **Zinc** is important for many biological reactions including the immune function, blood clotting, and wound healing – it can be found in oysters, crab, lean meats and poultry, pine nuts, cashew nuts, almonds, walnuts and chickpeas.

The wonders of juicing

For a nutrient-rich diet, I always recommend juicing to my patients. I have been juicing for many years and it gives me the energy to work the long hours my busy clinic demands. Studies have shown a correlation between drinking the juice of fruit and vegetables and a positive impact on the gut microbiota.[1]

I remember moving into my premises in 2002 and, having

moved my business and my home all in one go, I was exhausted. I could not find my juicer or anything else and I felt my energy plunge. I had to stay well and keep going to build up the centre and I could not afford to get ill.

The next day, I had a delivery of vegetables from my organic supplier, and having unpacked my juicer, I made a juice. Within 20 minutes of drinking this mixture my energy was restored and I felt I was back in the driving seat and able to continue. Over the years, I have combined various fruits and vegetables when making my juices, and here is one of my favourite recipes.

Vegetable juice recipe

Ingredients (when possible use organic produce)
- 1 apple
- 4-5 carrots
- ½ lettuce (not iceberg)
- 2 celery sticks
- ½ green pepper
- handful each of spinach, watercress and rocket
- small piece of ginger
- ¼ cucumber

The apple and ginger are to aid digestion; otherwise, the juice is too cold for the stomach.

Method
Wash all the ingredients and cut them so they can easily pass through the juicer.

Drink the juice at once, while it is fresh.

Blended vegetable juice (vegetable 'smoothie')

Some people don't have the time to juice so the following formula can be blended if time is an issue. However, personally, I don't find blending as beneficial as juicing. The difference between the two is that juicing separates the pulp of the ingredients from the juice, thereby a pure juice is extracted. Juicing also allows you to use more ingredients because the bulk of the fruit or vegetable is discarded; blending just mashes everything into a pulp which is very thick and harder to digest due to the high fibre content. Water is generally added to blended ingredients to make the smoothie easier to drink. The following recipe is suitable for a blender.

Ingredients

- handful each of spinach, rocket and watercress
- ¼ cucumber
- ½ apple
- small piece of ginger
- juice of ½ lemon

Method

Wash all the ingredients and cut them so they won't put too much stress on your blender.

Blend until the ingredients reach a smooth consistency and the liquid is pourable.

The mixture can be prepared fresh each day and watered down for drinking as and when required.

Finally

A healthy, balanced diet is the forerunner to maintaining good health. Therefore, it goes without saying, it should be the starting point in the treatment of all diseases.

I hope the information contained in this book will give you a greater understanding of the complexities of a Giardia infestation, its implications, and how to overcome it.

May good health be with you all.

References

Chapter 1: What is Giardia?

1. Public Health England. Giardia: Guidance and Data – the symptoms and epidemiology of giardiasis including travel-associated infections. 1 April 2014, updated 31 May 2018. www.gov.uk/guidance/giardia (Accessed 10 February 2019)
2. World Health Organization. The World Health Report 1996: Fighting Disease, Fostering Development. Geneva, Switzerland: WHO, 1996. https://www.who.int/whr/1996/en/ (Accessed 10 February 2019)
3. Adam RD. The biology of Giardia spp. *Microbiological Reviews* 1991; 55(4): 706–732.
4. Ford BJ. The discovery of Giardia. *Microscope* 2005; 53(4): 147–153.
5. Mitchell PD, Stern E, Tepper Y. Dysentery in the crusader kingdom of Jerusalem: an ELISA analysis of two medieval latrines in the City of Acre (Israel). *Journal of Archaeological Science* 2008; 35 (7): 1849–1853. doi:10.1016/j.jas.2007.11.017.
6. Nazer H. Giardiasis. *Medscape* 15 February 2016, updated 20 October 2018. http://emedicine.medscape.com/article/176718-overview (accessed 10 February 2019).
7. Monsters Inside Me S06E03. My Vacation from Hell. First broadcast 5 November 2015. USA. Discovery Channel. [YouTube video; 24.05–35.00] www.youtube.com/watch?v=Ln81ebbCa0s (Accessed 17 November 2016).
8. Olson BE, Olson ME, Wallis PM (Eds). *Giardia: The Cosmopolitan Parasite*. Wallingford, UK: CABI International; 2002: page 5.

9. Parulekar SG. Ultrasound evaluation of common bile duct size. *Radiology* 1979; 133 (3Pt1): 703–707.

10. Bemrick WJ. Some perspectives on the transmission of giardiasis. In: Erlandsen SL, Meyer EA (Eds) *Giardia and Giardiasis: Biology, Pathogenesis and Epidemiology.* New York, US: Plenum Press 1984; pages 379–400.

Chapter 2: Getting a diagnosis

1. Public Health England. Giardia: Guidance and Data – the symptoms and epidemiology of giardiasis including travel-associated infections. 1 April 2014, updated 31 May 2018. www.gov.uk/guidance/giardia (Accessed 10 February 2019)

2. Minetti C, Chalmers RM, Beeching NJ, Probert C, Lamden K. Giardiasis. *BMJ* 2016: 335. doi.org/10.1136/bmj.i5369

3. Hisham Nazer. Giardiasis Workup. *MedScape* Updated 1 October 2018. http://emedicine.medscape.com/article/176718-workup (Accessed 10 February 2019)

4. Tidy C, Bonsall A. Irritable Bowel Syndrome. Patient Platform Limited, England & Wales. 2 July 2017. https://patient.info/health/irritable-bowel-syndrome-leaflet (Accessed 10 February 2019)

Chapter 3: Checking for Giardia

1. Di Prisco CM, Hagel I, Lynch NR, Jiménez JC, Rojas R, Gil M, Mata E. Association between giardiasis and allergy. *Ann Allergy Asthma Immunol* 1998; 81(3): 261-265. (PubMed)

2. Overeem MMA, Verhagen LM, Hermans PWM, del Nogal B, Márquez Sánchez A, Martinez Acevedo N, Ramirez Murga R, Roelfsema J, Pinelli E, de Waard JH. Recurrent wheezing is associated with intestinal protozoan infections in Warao Amerindian children in Venezuela: a cross-sectional survey. *BMC – Infectious Disease* 2014; 14: 293. doi: 10.1186/1471-2334-14-293

3. Mørch K, Hanevik K, Rivenes AC, Bødtker JE, Næss H, Stubhaug B, Wensaas K-A, Rortveit G, Eide GE, Hausken T, Langeland N. Chronic fatigue syndrome 5 years after giardiasis: differential diagnoses, characteristics and natural course *BMC*

– *Gastroenterology* 2013; 13: 28 www.biomedcentral.com/1471-230X/13/28

4. Khan WU, Sellen DW. Zinc supplementation in the management of diarrhoea. World Health Organization, 2011. www.who.int/elena/titles/bbc/zinc_diarrhoea/en/ (Accessed 28 Feb 2019)

5. Klotz SA, Penn CC, Negvesky GJ, Butrus SI. Fungal and parasitic infections of the eye. *Clinical Microbiol Rev* 2000; 13(4): 662-685. doi:10.1128/CMR.13.4.662-685.2000

6. Simsek Z, Zeyrek FY, Kurcer MA. Effect of Giardia infection on growth and psychomotor development of children aged 0-5 years. *Journal of Tropical Pediatrics* 2004; 50(2): 90-93. https://pdfs.semanticscholar.org/a60f/1b0d81482a426d431b355aa421cb2dd56907.pdf

7. Halliez MCM, Buret AG. Extra-intestinal and long term consequences of *Giardia duodenalis* infections. *World Journal of Gastroenterology* 2013; 19(47): 8974–8985. doi: 10.3748/wjg.v19.i47.8974: PMCID: PMC3870550

8. Carlson DW, Finger DR. Beaver fever arthritis. *Journal of Clinical Rheumatology* 2004;10: 86–88. (www.ncbi.nlm.nih.gov/pubmed/17043473)

9. Wilhelm RE. Urticaria associated with giardiasis lamblia. *Journal of Allergy* 1957; 28(4): 351-353. DOI: org/10.1016/0021-8707(57)90047-3

Chapter 4: Gut reactions

1. Coeliac UK. About coeliac disease. www.coeliac.org.uk/coeliac-disease/about-coeliac-disease-and-dermatitis-herpetiformis/ (Accessed 28 February 2019)

2. Gujral N, Freeman HJ, Thomson ABR. Celiac disease: Prevalence, diagnosis, pathogenesis and treatment. *World Journal of Gastroenterology* 2012; 18(42): 6036-6059.

3. Carroccio A, Cavataio F, Montalto G, Paparo F, Troncone R, Iacono G. Treatment of giardiasis reverses 'active' coeliac disease to 'latent' coeliac disease. *European Journal of Gastroenterology & Hepatology* 2001; 13(9): 1101–1105.

4. Wolfe MS. Giardiasis. *JAMA* 1975; 233(13): 1362–1365. doi: 10.1001/jama.1975.03260130020014.

5. Pettoello Mantovani M, Guandalini S, Ecuba P, Corvino C, di Martino L. Lactose malabsorption in children with symptomatic

Giardia lamblia infection: feasibility of yogurt supplementation. *Journal of Pediatric Gastroenterology and Nutrition* 1989; 9(3): 295–300.

6.   Fuller R. Probiotics in human medicine. *Gut* 1991; 32(4): 439–442. PMCID: PMC1379087

7.   Guarner F, Malagelada J-R. Gut flora in health and disease. *The Lancet* 2003: 8; 360.

8.   Galland L. Leaky gut syndromes: breaking the vicious cycle. *Foundation for Integrated Medicine* 2007. http://mdheal.org/ leakygut.htm (Accessed 10 February 2019).

9.   Cordingley FT, Crawford GPM. Giardia infection causes vitamin B12 deficiency. *Australian & New Zealand Journal of Medicine* 1986; 16(1): 78–79.

Chapter 5: Giardia and stress

1.   Selye H. Stress and the general adaptation syndrome. *British Medical Journal* 1950; 1(4667): 1383-1392. www.ncbi.nlm.nih.gov/ pmc/articles/PMC2038162/Wikipedia. (Accessed 17 February 2019) and Hans Selye.https://en.wikipedia.org/wiki/Hans_Selye (Last updated 10 February 2019; accessed 10 February 2019)

2.   Segerstrom SC, Miller GE. Psychological stress and the human immune system: a meta-analytic study of 30 years of inquiry. *Psychol Bull* 2004; 130(4): 601-630. doi: 10.1037/0033-2909.130.4.601

3.   Anxiety UK. Anxiety conditions. 2018 www.anxietyuk.org.uk/ get-help/anxiety-information/ (Accessed 10 February 2019)

4.   Stormorken E, Jason LA, Kirkevold M. From good health to illness with post-infectious fatigue syndrome: a qualitative study of adults' experiences of the illness trajectory. *BCM: Family Practice* 2017; 18: 49. doi.org/10.1186/s12875-017-0614-4

Chapter 6: Giardia and our natural defence barriers

1.   Allain T, Amat CB, Motta J-P, Buret AG. Interactions of Giardia sp. with the intestinal barrier: epithelium, mucus and microbiota. *Tissue Barriers* 2017; 5(1): e1274354. www.ncbi.nlm.nih.gov/pmc/ articles/PMC5362998/#!po=21.8447

2.   AMNH. Secret World Inside You Exhibition. Building your microbiome from birth. American Museum of Natural History. www.amnh.org/exhibitions/the-secret-world-inside-you/building-your-microbiome-from-birth/ (Accessed 28 Feb 2019)

3.   Yassour M, Vatanen T, Siljander H, Hamalainene A-M, et al. Natural history of the infant gut microbiome and impact of antibiotic treatments on strain-level and diversity. *Sci Trans Med* 2016; 8(343): 343ra81. doi: 10.1126/scitranslmed.aad0917

4.   Yang I, Corwin EJ, Brennan PA, Jordan S, et al. The Infant Microbiome: Implications for Infant Health and Neurocognitive Development. *Nursing Research* 2016; 65(1): 76-88. doi: 10.1097/NNR.0000000000000133

5.   Kutty PK. Breastfeeding and risk of parasitic infection – a review. *Asian Pacific Journal of Tropical Biomedicine* 2014; 4(11): 847-858. doi.org/10.12980/APJTB.4.201414B355

6.   Higdon J, Drake VJ, Angela G, Delage B, Carr AC, Michels AJ. Vitamin C. Linus Pauling Institute, Oregon State University. 2000-2019 https://lpi.oregonstate.edu/mic/vitamins/vitamin-C (Accessed 10 February 2019)

Chapter 7: Allergies

1.   Li E, Zhou P, Petrin Z, Singer SM. Mast Cell-Dependent Control of *Giardia lamblia* Infections in Mice. *Infect Immun* 2004; 72(11): 6642–6649. doi: 10.1128/IAI.72.11.6642-6649.2004

2.   Allergy UK. Allergy statistics. www.allergyuk.org/allergy-statistics/allergy-statistics (Accessed 28 Feb 2019)

3.   Di Prisco MC, Hagel I, Lynch NR, Jiménez JC, Rojas R, Gil M, Mata E. Association between giardiasis and allergy. *Ann Allergy Asthma Immunol* 1998; 81(3): 261-265. (www.ncbi.nlm.nih.gov/pubmed/9759805)

4.   Allergy UK. Allergy Statistics. Allergy UK. www.allergyuk.org/allergy-statistics/allergy-statistics (Accessed 28 Feb 2019)

5.   Galland L. Intestinal protozoan infestation and systemic illness. *Foundation for Integrated Medicine* http://mdheal.org/articles/word2/intestinalprotozoan2.htm (Accessed 10 February 2019).

6.   NHS Inform. Corticosteroids. www.nhsinform.scot/tests-and-treatments/medicines-and-medical-aids/types-of-medicine/

corticosteroids (Last updated 5 February 2019; accessed 10 February 2019)

7.   Olson BE, Olson ME, Wallis PM. *Giardia - the Cosmopolitan Parasite.* CABI, Wallingford, Oxon, UK; 2002.

8.   Nenoff P. Giardia lamblia – cause of urticaria and pruritus or accidental association? *Hautarzt* 2006; 57(6): 521-522. DOI: 10.1007/ s00105-005-0959-9

9.   McKnight JT, Tietze PE. Dermatologic manifestations of giardiasis. (PMID:1496900) *J Am Board Fam Pract* 1992; 5(4): 425-428.

Chapter 8: The gallbladder connection

1.   MacPhee L, Walker BS. Intestinal giardiasis in New England, with notes on its pathogenicity and symptomatology. *American Journal of Digestive Diseases and Nutrition* 1934; 1(10): 768-773. https://link. springer.com/article/10.1007%2FBF02999602?LI=true

2.   University of Edinburgh. Gallbladder surgery risks studied. University of Edinburgh; 13 April 2016. www.ed.ac.uk/news/ all-news/gallbladder-280612 (Accessed 28 Feb 2019)

Chapter 9: The pancreas connection

1.   Ding M, Satija A, Bhupathiraju SN, Hu Y, et al. Association of coffee consumption with total and cause-specific mortality in three large prospective cohorts. *Circulation* 2015; 132(24): 2305-2315. doi: 10.1161/CIRCULATIONAHA.115.017341

2.   Nilsson AC, Johansson-Boll EV, Björck IME. Increased gut hormones and insulin sensitivity index following a 3-d intervention with a barley kernel-based product: a randomised cross-over study in healthy middle-aged subjects. *British Journal of Nutrition* 2015; 114(06): 899. DOI: 10.1017/S0007114515002524

3.   Ramirez CE, Hui N, Yu C, Gamboa JL, Luther JM, Brown NJ, Shibao CA. Treatment with Sildenafil improves insulin sensitivity in prediabetes: A randomized, controlled trial. *Journal of Clinical Endocrinology & Metabolism* 2015; jc: 3415 DOI: 10.1210/jc.2015-3415)

4.   Volpe KD. Viagra improves insulin sensitivity in people with prediabetes. EndocrineWeb. www.endocrineweb.com/

professional/pre-diabetes/viagra-improves-insulin-sensitivity-people-prediabetes (Updated 30 April 2018; accessed 28 Feb 2019)
5. Diabetes Research Foundation: Type 1 Diabetes Facts and Figures. Input: JDRF. https://jdrf.org.uk/information-support/about-type-1-diabetes/facts-and-figures/ (Accessed 28 Feb 2019)
6. Native Remedies. The Pancreas. https://www.nativeremedies.com/ailment/symptoms-of-pancreas-problems.html (Accessed 10 February 2019)
7. Schwingshacki L, Hoffmann G. Adherence to Mediterranean diet and risk of cancer: an updated systematic review and meta-analysis of observational studies. *Cancer Medicine* 2015; 4(12): 1933-1947. www.ncbi.nlm.nih.gov/pmc/articles/PMC5123783/
8. Lloyd C, Smith J, Weinger K. Stress and diabetes: A review of the links. *Diabetes Spectrum* 2005; 18(2): 121-127. doi.org/10.2337/diaspect.18.2.121

Chapter 10: Prevention

1. Jarroll EL, Bingham AK, Meyer EA. Effect of chlorine on Giardia lamblia cyst viability. *Applied Environmental Microbiology* 1981; 41(2): 483-487. www.ncbi.nlm.nih.gov/pmc/articles/PMC243720/
2. Gray SF, Gunnell DJ, Peters TJ. Risk factors for giardiasis: a case-control study in Avon and Somerset. *Epidemiol Infect* 1994; 113(1): 95-102. www.ncbi.nlm.nih.gov/pubmed/8062884
3. CDC. Food and Water Safety. The Centers for Disease Control and Prevention; Atlanta, USA
https://wwwnc.cdc.gov/travel/page/food-water-safety
4. London School of Hygiene and Tropical Medicine. Contamination of UK mobile phones and hands revealed. 14 October 2011. www.lshtm.ac.uk/newsevents/news/2011/mobilephones.html (Accessed 10 February 2019)
5. World Health Organization. Hand Hygiene – why, how and when. August 2009. www.who.int/gpsc/5may/Hand_Hygiene_Why_How_and_When_Brochure.pdf (Accessed 10 February 2019)
6. CDC. Parasites: Giardia - Prevention & Control. Centers for Disease Control and Prevention, Atlanta, USA. www.cdc.gov/parasites/giardia/prevention-control-general-public.html

Chapter 11: Treating giardiasis

1. Mayo Clinic. Giardia infection (giardiasis). www.mayoclinic.org/diseases-conditions/giardiainfection/symptoms-causes/syc-20372786 (Accessed 10 February 2019)
2. NHS. Metronidazole. 6 December 2018. www.nhs.uk/medicines/metronidazole/ (Accessed 10 February 2019)
3. Carter ER, Nabarro LE, Hedley L, Chiodini PL. Nitroimidazole-refractory giardiasis Nitroimidazole-refractory giardiasis: a growing problem requiring rational solutions. *Clinical Microbiology and Infection* 2018; 24(1): 37-42. doi.org/10.1016/j.cmi.2017.05.028
4. Taylor GD, Wenman WM, Tyrrell DL. Combined metronidazole and quinacrine hydrochloride therapy for chronic giardiasis. *CAMJ* 1987; 136(11): 1179-1180. www.ncbi.nlm.nih.gov/pmc/articles/PMC1492164/
5. World Health Organization. WHO Monograph on good agricultural and collection practices for Artemisia annua L. WHO, 2006. www.who.int/medicines/publications/traditional/ArtemisiaMonograph.pdf
6. World Health Organization. Antimalarial Drug Combination Therapy – report of a WHO technical consultation. WHO, 2001. https://apps.who.int/iris/bitstream/handle/10665/66952/WHO_CDS_RBM_2001.35.pdf;jsessionid=89D69DDFAB72A9AC1755CE755D5B72CB?sequence=1
7. Loo CSN, Lam NSK, Yu D, Su X, Lu F. Artemisinin and its derivatives in treating protozoan infections beyond malaria. *Pharmacol Reseearch* 2017; 117: 192-217. doi: 10.1016/j.phrs.2016.11.012

Chapter 12: Healing through energy fields

1. Wikipedia. Schumann resonances. https://en.wikipedia.org/wiki/Schumann_resonances
2. Einthoven W. The string galvanometer and the measurement of the action currents of the heart. Nobel Lecture, 11 December 1925. www.nobelprize.org/uploads/2018/06/einthoven-lecture.pdf
3. Rubik B, Muesham D. Biofield science and healing – history,

terminology and concepts. *Global Advances Health Med* 2015; 4(Suppl): 8-14. www.ncbi.nlm.nih.gov/pmc/articles/ PMC4654789/

4. Karagulla S, Kunz D. *The Chakras and the Human Energy Fields.* Wheaton, Ill, US: Theosophical Publishing House, 1989.

Appendix I: Herbs

1. Khan A, Qadir SS, Khan NK, Anderson RA; Cloves improve glucose, cholesterol and triglycerides of people with type 2 diabetes mellitus. *The FASEB Journal* 7 March 2006 www.fasebj. org/doi/abs/10.1096/fasebj.20.5.A990-b (Accessed 28 Feb 2019)

2. Lauwaet T, Andersen Y, Van de Ven L, Eckmann L, Gillin FD. Rapid detachment of Giardia lamblia trophozoites as a mechanism of antimicrobial action of the isoflavone formononetin. *Journal of Antimicrob Chemother* 2010 March; 65(3): 531–534.

Appendix III: Living without gluten

1. Commission Implementing Regulation (EU) No 828/2014 of 30 July 2014 on the requirements for the provision of information to consumers on the absence or reduced presence of gluten in food. EU Commission – EUR-Lex. https://eur-lex.europa.eu/legal-content/EN/TXT/?uri=CELEX:32014R0828

2. Coeliac UK. Live well gluten free. Grains. www.coeliac.org. uk/gluten-free-diet-and-lifestyle/gf-diet/grains/ (Accessed 10 February 2019)

Appendix IV: Maintaining a healthy gut microbiome

1. Henning SM, Yang J, Shao P, et al. Health benefit of vegetable/fruit juice-based diet: role of microbiome. *Scientific Reports* 2017; 7(1): 2167. DOI: 10.1038/s41598-017-02200-6

Index

abdominal distension, 28
Achillea millefolium, 141
acidity
  duodenum, 9
  jejunum, 9
  stomach, 7, 96–97, 98
adaptation (stress response), 44
Agropyron repens (couchgrass), 133
alarm reaction, 44
Alison's story, 50–52
alkaline environment, 7, 83, 97, 98
allergy, 4–5, 26, 63–73
  food, 39, 69–71
  skin, 71–72
allopathic approach (with antiprotozoals - also referred to as antimicrobials), 8, 106–109
anaphylactic shock, 70
angioedema, 71–72
animals, 95–96
aniseed, 130
Ann's story, 114–115
anogenital area and sexual activity, 96
antibiotics (antibacterials), ix-x

antibiotics (antiprotozoals - also referred to as antimicrobials), 8, 106–109
antibodies
  coeliac disease and, 36, 37
  food allergy and, 86
  Giardia and, 2, 8
antimalarials, 10, 108, 109–110, 110–111
anus, genital contamination with cysts from, 96
apathy, 26
Artemesia annua see wormwood
artemisinin, 110
artichoke, globe, 135
asthma, 26, 64–65
aura (light body), 118, 119, 120
autoimmune disorder
  coeliac disease as, 27, 34, 35
  diabetes type 1 as, 88, 89
Azadirachta indica, 137

babies *see* infants
bacteria (gut)
  beneficial/healthy/friendly, 54, 55–56, 101–102
  harmful, 54, 57, 100
  see also microbiome

Index

bad breath, 27
barberry, 130
base chakra, 122
Beardall, Alan (Dr), 21
Becky's story, 59–61
Berberis vulgaris (barberry), 130
biliary tract, 75
    bile duct (and its blockage),
        8, 9, 30, 74, 83
    see also gallbladder
biofields, 118
biofilms, 55
birth and microbiome
        formation, 56–57
boldo, 130–131
bowel habit/movement
        changes, 17, 18, 27
    see also gut; inflammatory
        bowel disease; irritable
        bowel syndrome
breastfeeding, 57, 58
breath
    bad, 27
    shortness, 29
Brennan, Barbara Ann (Dr), 119,
        121
bruxism, 29–30
buckwheat, 147

caesarean birth and the
        microbiome, 57
Calendula officinalis (marigold),
        137
Capsicum minimum (cayenne;
        chilli), 131
Carol's story, 76–80
case histories
    preface, ix-xii
    chapter 1, 5–6, 10–12
    chapter 2, 15, 22–23
    chapter 3, 32–33

    chapter 4, 35, 37–38, 40–41
    chapter 5, 42–43, 50–52
    chapter 6, 59–61
    chapter 7, 65–66, 72–73
    chapter 8, 76–80
    chapter 9, 85–91
    chapter 10, 97, 103–104
    chapter 11, 110–111, 114–115
cayenne, chilli, 131
cell (mobile) phones, 69, 98
centaury, 131
cereal grains, gluten-free,
        145–150
chakras, 121–123, 123–124, 124
chamomile, German, 131–132
chaparral, 132
chi (prana; chi), 119, 120
chia, 150
children, 58–59
    hygiene, 58, 99
    lactose intolerances, 38–39
    see also infants
chill(s), 27
chilli cayenne, 131
Chionanthes virginicus (fringe
        tree), 134
cholecystectomy (gallbladder
        removal), 75–80
Christopher's story, 97
chronic fatigue syndrome, 27
cinnamon, 132
close contact with infected
        persons, 94–95
clove, 132–133
clover, red, 101, 139
cobblestone appearance, 7
coeliac disease, 27, 34, 35–38,
        150
    see also gluten
Collinsonia canadensis (stone
        root), 140

Commiphora molmol (myrrh), 137

comprehensive parasitology stool test, 15, 16–17, 32

constipation, 27

corn, 146

cortisol, 44, 46, 48

couchgrass, 133

cough, chronic, 27

couscous, 148–149

cramps, stomach, 29

creamy-coloured/yellow stools, 30

creosote bush, 132

Crohn's disease, 18

crown chakra, 122

Cynara scolymu (globe artichoke), 135

cysts, 3, 9
   biliary system, 74, 83
   pancreatic duct, 83
   sexual activity and, 96

defences (against Giardia), 54–62
   immune system *see* immune system
   natural, 54–62

depression, 28

diabetes, 28
   type 1, 83–84, 85–91
   type 2, 8, 83, 84

diagnosis, 14–25, 32

diarrhoea, 3, 4, 28
   case stories, 10, 11, 12, 22, 35, 42, 43, 76, 77, 79, 103, 110, 111, 115

diet, 144–158
   healthy, 84, 151–154
   poor, 61–62
   see also food

digestive system *see* gut

drinking water, 93–94, 95, 99–100

drugs *see* antibiotics; antimalarials

duodenum, 8, 9, 74, 75, 76, 83

Dusan, Vilem (Dr), 1

echinacea, 133

elder, 134

electrocardiogram, 118

electroencephalogram, 118

Ely, John (Dr), 62

emotional response to stress, 49

energy fields and systems, 113, 117–125

enzyme-linked immunosorbent assay (ELISA), 15, 16, 32, 48, 81

Erythraea centarium (centaury), 131

Eunonymous atropapeurins (wahoo), 141

Eupatorium purpureum (gravel root), 135–136

exhaustion (in stress), 44

eye problems, 28

faeces *see* stools

family
   close contact with infected members of, 94–95
   stress and family occasions, 43

farm animals, 95

fatigue *see* apathy; chronic fatigue syndrome; exhaustion; lethargy; tiredness; weakness

feeding stage *see* trophozoites

fermented foods, 151–154

ferritin levels, 38
fever, 27
filters, water, 100
Flagyl *see* metronidazole
flight-or-fight response, 44, 45, 46
folate/folic acid, 155
food, raw and partially cooked, 95
see also diet
food allergy, 39, 69–71
food intolerances, 6–7, 28, 69–71
gluten, 6, 36, 150
lactose, 38–39
foreign travel (travel abroad), 10, 14, 106
friends, close contact with, 94–95
fringe tree, 134
fruits and vegetables, juicing, 155–157

Galega officinalis (goat's rue), 135
gallbladder, 30, 74–81
checklist, 80–81
removal, 75–80
role, 75
stones, 9, 75, 76, 77
gastrointestinal tract *see* gut
Gemma (author's friend), xi
general adaptation syndrome, 44
genital contamination with cysts from anus, 96
gentian, 134
German chamomile, 131–132
Giard, Alfred (Professor), 1
Giardia (basics about), 1–13
checking for, 26–33
defence against *see* defences
diagnosis, 14–25, 32

life cycle, 7–9
prevention of infection, 92–105
stress and *see* stress
symptoms of giardiasis *see* symptoms
testing for, 14–25, 32
transmission routes, 93–96
treatment of infection *see* treatment
ginger, 135
gliadin, 36, 70
globe artichoke, 135
glucagon, 84
glucose, blood (blood sugar), 83, 84, 85, 86, 90
glucose-ascorbate-antagonism theory, 62
gluten, 144–150
diets without, 34, 35, 36, 37, 144–150
intolerance, 6, 36, 150
see also coeliac disease
goat's rue, 135
Goodheart, George J (Dr), 20
grains, gluten-free, 145–150
gravel root, 135–136
growth retardation, 28
gut (digestive/gastrointestinal system incl. stomach/intestine)
microbiome, 54, 55–57
symptoms and illnesses
case stories, ix, x, xi, 4, 27, 28, 29, 34–41
historical perspectives, 2
see also bowel habit; cramps; duodenum; inflammatory bowel disease; irritable bowel syndrome; stomach
Gymnema sylvestre, 139

halitosis (bad breath), 27
hand washing, 92, 94, 96, 99,
    101
hay fever, 67
headaches, 28
heart chakra, 122
herbs and plants, 111–114,
    129–141
    author's early experiences,
        xiii–xiv
    sprays, 59, 90, 113–114, 120,
        123–125
histamine, 63, 67, 70, 71
historical perspectives, 1–2
hives (urticaria), 71
holidays and stress, 43
host–parasite interactions, 2–3
hydrangea, 136
hygiene, 95
    children, 58, 99
    farm animals, 95
    hand (and washing hands),
        92, 94, 96, 98–99, 101

iced water, 95
immune system, 73, 102
    allergy and, 63–64
    coeliac disease and, 35–36
    compromised, 2, 48, 53, 73,
        102
    stress and, 45–46, 45–46
    trophozoite avoiding
        recognition by, 8
    vitamins and minerals,
        154–155
    see also autoimmune
        disorder
Indian arrow tree (wahoo), 141
infants (babies)
    breastfeeding, 57, 58
    nappies, 94

newborns, microbiome
    formation, 56–57
inflammatory bowel disease
    (IBD), testing, 18–19
insulin, 82–83, 84
    administration, 82–83, 86,
        87, 88, 89, 90
    resistance, 83, 85, 87, 91
intestine see bowel; gut
iron, 155
irritable bowel syndrome (IBS),
    14, 15, 17–18, 28
    case stories, 15, 23, 35, 42,
        60, 76, 97, 111
    testing for, 17–18

James's story, 35
Jane's story, 10–11, 42–43
jejunum, 8, 9
joint pain, 29
juicing, 155–157
Julia's story, 11–12

kefir, 152–153
kinesiology
    applied (AK), 15, 19–22
    clinical (CK), 21
Kirlian photography, 118
Koten, Susan, in case stories,
        xi–x, 5–6, 11–12, 15, 23–24,
        32–33, 35, 42, 51–52,
        60–61, 65–66, 72–73, 87,
        89–90, 97, 104, 115
Kriya cleansing programme, 68

lactose intolerances, 38–39
Larium (mefloquine), 10,
    110–111
Larrea tridentate (chaparral), 132
laundry, 101
Laura's story, 5–6

lavender, 136
leaky gut syndrome, 39
Leeuwenhoek, Antony van, 1
leptandra, 136
lethargy, 28–29
life cycle of Giardia, 7–9
light body (aura), 118, 119, 120

malaria and antimalarials, 10,
    108, 109–110, 110–111
marigold, 137
Mary's story, 40–41
mast cells, 63
Matricaria recutita (German
    chamomile), 131–132
Maureen's story, 72–73
Mediterranean diet, 84
mefloquine (Larium), 10,
    110–111
Melanie's story, 88–91
Mentha piperita, 138–139
metronidazole (Flagyl), 107
    alternative drugs to, 108
    case stories, 10, 11, 40, 111,
        114
microbiome (flora), 54, 55–57,
    151–158
    healthy, 55–57, 151–158
    see also bacteria
millet, 148
minerals, 154, 155
mobile phones, 69, 98
mould allergy, 69
mucus
    barrier function in gut, 55
    in stools, 29
muscles
    pain, 29
    testing, 15, 19–22
myrrh, 137

nappies, 94
nausea, 29
neem tree, 137
nettle, 138
newborns, microbiome
    formation, 56–57
Nikki's story, ix–x
noisy intestine, 29
nutrition *see* diet; food

offensive-smelling stools, 29
old man's beard (fringe tree),
    134
omeprazole, 96, 97, 98
ova and parasite test (stool),
    16

Page, Nikki, story, ix–x
pain, muscle and joint, 29
pancreas, 82–91
    maintaining health of, 84–85
Parietaria officinalis, 138
patient stories *see* case histories
Pauling, Linus, 62
pellitory of the wall (*Parietaria
    officinalis*), 138
Penny's story, 37–38
peppermint (*Mentha piperita*),
    138–139
perennial allergic rhinitis, 67
periploca of the wood
    (*Gymnema sylvestre*), 139
pets, 95–96
Peumus boldo (boldo), 130–131
Pimpinella anisum (aniseed),
    130
pollen, 67
popcorn, home-made, 146
prana (qi; chi), 119, 120
pregnancy, 57–58
prevention, 92–105

probiotics
    foods containing, 152, 153
    in gut, 56, 102, 151
proton pump inhibitors, 96–97
protozoon, definition, 7
public water coolers, 93–94
    public buildings, 95

qi (chi; prana), 119, 120
Qing-hao see wormwood
quinacrine, 108–109
quinoa, 147

Rainbow diet, 84
red clover, 101, 139
resistance (stress response), 44
rhinitis, allergic, 67
rice, 145–146
Riordan, Dr, xi
risk (of Giardia infection),
    understanding, 98–99
routes of transmission, 93–96

sacral chakra, 122
Sally's story, 110–111
Sambucus nigra (elder), 134
sauerkraut, 153–154
Schumann Cavity Resonance,
    117
selenium, 155
Selye, Hans, 44
sexual activity, 96
sinuses and allergy, 68–69
skin problems, 6, 29
    allergic, 71–72
sleep problems, 5–6, 29
smelly stools, 29
smoothie, vegetable, 157
solar plexus chakra, 122
Sophie's story, 22–23
sorghum, 149

spindle tree (wahoo), 141
sprays (herbal), 59, 90, 113–114,
    120, 123–125
SQID (superconducting
    quantum interference
    device), 118
steamed coconut rice, 145–146
steroid hormones and stress, 44
stomach
    acidity, 7, 96–97
    cramps, 29
    see also abdominal
        distension; gut
stone(s)
    gallbladder, 9, 75, 76, 77
    urinary tract, 142
stone root, 140
stools (faeces)
    animal, human infection
        from, 86
    mucus in, 29
    smelly, 29
    tests, 15–17, 32
    yellow / creamy-coloured,
        30
stories *see* case histories
stress, 42–53
    defining, 44–45
    diabetes and, 84
    immune system and, 45–46
string test, 15, 16
subtle bodies, 119
sugar
    blood (blood glucose), 83,
        84, 85, 86, 90
    dietary, 61–62
superconducting quantum
    interference device
    (SQID), 118
surfaces, dirty, 94
sweating, 29

sweet wormwood / sweet Annie
  see wormwood
symptoms (giardiasis), 4–7,
  26–33
  checklist, 31, 80–81
  gallbladder problems, 80–81
  gut *see* gut
  recognising, 4–7
symptoms (other conditions)
  allergies, 39, 63, 64, 67, 69, 70
  coeliac disease, 36
  food intolerance, 70
  gallbladder problems,
    80–81
  IBD, 18
  IBS, 17
  leaky gut syndrome, 39
  stress, recognising, 46–48
  vitamin B12 deficiency, 39
Syzigium aromaticum (clove),
  132–133

teeth grinding, 29–30
teff, 149–150
tests (diagnostic), 14–25, 32
third-eye chakra, 122
threat response, 45–46
throat chakra, 122
thuja, 140
thymus, 141
tinidazole (Tindamax), 108, 114
tiredness, 78
  see also apathy; chronic
    fatigue syndrome;
    exhaustion; lethargy;
    weakness
tissue transglutaminase (tTG)
  IgA test, 36, 37
toilets
  hand washing, 94, 101
  pets drinking water from, 96

Tom's story, 65–66
Tony's story, 103–104
tooth grinding, 29–30
transmission routes, 93–96
travel abroad, 10, 14, 106
treatment, 106–125
  herbs *see* herbs and plants
Trifolium pratense (red clover),
  101, 139
trophozoites (feeding stage),
  7–9
  biliary system, 74–75, 81,
    83
  pancreatic duct, 83

ulcerative colitis, 18
urinary tract stones, 142
Urtica dioica (nettle), 138
urticaria, 71

vaginal birth and the
  microbiome, 56–57
van Leeuwenhoek, Antony, 1
vegetables and fruit, juicing,
  155–157
vibrations and vibrational
  frequency, 117, 121, 123,
  124
villi, 34, 36, 38
vitamin A, 154
vitamin B9, 155
vitamin B12 deficiency, 26–27,
  39–41
vitamin C, 62, 154–155
vitamin D, 38
vitamin E, 155
vomiting, 30

wahoo, 141
washing hands, 92, 94, 96,
  98–99, 101

water (ingestion)
   dirty water, 93
   drinking water, 93–94, 95,
     99–100
   iced water, 95
weakness, 30
weight loss, 39
wheat allergy, 70–71
white fringe tree, 134
Willow Herbal Centre, 5, 60, 72,
     87, 97
wind, 30
work and stress, 42–43
wormwood (*Artemesia annua*;
     sweet annie; sweet
     wormwood; *Qing-hao*), 75,
     109–110, 112–113, 140

case stories, xii, 6, 10, 11, 12,
   24, 32, 37, 38, 40, 41, 59,
   60, 72, 74, 79, 87, 93, 111
   infusion, 112–113
   pregnancy and, 57–58

yarrow, 141
yellow / creamy-coloured stools,
   30
yoghurt and lactose
   intolerances, 38–39

zinc, 155
Zingiber officinalis (ginger), 135